Emergency Neuro-Otology: Diagnosis and Management of Acute Dizziness and Vertigo

Editors

DAVID E. NEWMAN-TOKER
KEVIN A. KERBER
WILLIAM J. MEURER
RODNEY OMRON
JONATHAN A. EDLOW

NEUROLOGIC CLINICS

www.neurologic.theclinics.com

Consulting Editor
RANDOLPH W. EVANS

August 2015 • Volume 33 • Number 3

1600 John F. Kennedy Boulevard • Suite 1800 • Philadelphia, Pennsylvania, 19103-2899

http://www.theclinics.com

NEUROLOGIC CLINICS Volume 33, Number 3
August 2015 ISSN 0733-8619, ISBN-13: 978-0-323-39346-1

Editor: Lauren Boyle
Developmental editor: Donald Mumford

© **2015 Elsevier Inc. All rights reserved.**

This periodical and the individual contributions contained in it are protected under copyright by Elsevier, and the following terms and conditions apply to their use:

Photocopying
Single photocopies of single articles may be made for personal use as allowed by national copyright laws. Permission of the Publisher and payment of a fee is required for all other photocopying, including multiple or systematic copying, copying for advertising or promotional purposes, resale, and all forms of document delivery. Special rates are available for educational institutions that wish to make photocopies for non-profit educational classroom use. For information on how to seek permission visit www.elsevier.com/permissions or call: (+44) 1865 843830 (UK)/(+1) 215 239 3804 (USA).

Derivative Works
Subscribers may reproduce tables of contents or prepare lists of articles including abstracts for internal circulation within their institutions. Permission of the Publisher is required for resale or distribution outside the institution. Permission of the Publisher is required for all other derivative works, including compilations and translations (please consult www.elsevier.com/permissions).

Electronic Storage or Usage
Permission of the Publisher is required to store or use electronically any material contained in this periodical, including any article or part of an article (please consult www.elsevier.com/permissions). Except as outlined above, no part of this publication may be reproduced, stored in a retrieval system or transmitted in any form or by any means, electronic, mechanical, photocopying, recording or otherwise, without prior written permission of the Publisher.

Notice
No responsibility is assumed by the Publisher for any injury and/or damage to persons or property as a matter of products liability, negligence or otherwise, or from any use or operation of any methods, products, instructions or ideas contained in the material herein. Because of rapid advances in the medical sciences, in particular, independent verification of diagnoses and drug dosages should be made.

Although all advertising material is expected to conform to ethical (medical) standards, inclusion in this publication does not constitute a guarantee or endorsement of the quality or value of such product or of the claims made of it by its manufacturer.

Neurologic Clinics (ISSN 0733-8619) is published quarterly by Elsevier Inc., 360 Park Avenue South, New York, NY 10010–1710. Months of issue are February, May, August, and November. Periodicals postage paid at New York, NY, and additional mailing offices. Subscription prices are $300.00 per year for US individuals, $517.00 per year for US institutions, $145.00 per year for US students, $375.00 per year for Canadian individuals, $627.00 per year for Canadian institutions, $415.00 per year for international individuals, $627.00 per year for international institutions, and $210.00 for Canadian and foreign students/residents. To receive student/resident rate, orders must be accompanied by name of affiliated institution, date of term, and the *signature* of program/residency coordinator on institution letterhead. Orders will be billed at individual rate until proof of status is received. Foreign air speed delivery is included in all *Clinics* subscription prices. All prices are subject to change without notice. **POSTMASTER:** Send address changes to *Neurologic Clinics*, Elsevier Health Sciences Division, Subscription Customer Service, 3251 Riverport Lane, Maryland Heights, MO 63043. **Customer Service: Telephone: 1-800-654-2452 (U.S. and Canada); 314-447-8871 (outside U.S. and Canada). Fax: 314-447-8029. E-mail: journalscustomerservice-usa@elsevier.com (for print support); journalsonlinesupport-usa@elsevier.com (for online support).**

Reprints. For copies of 100 or more of articles in this publication, please contact the Commercial Reprints Department, Elsevier Inc., 360 Park Avenue South, New York, New York, 10010-1710; Tel.: +1-212-633-3874; Fax: +1-212-633-3820, and E-mail: reprints@elsevier.com.

Neurologic Clinics is also published in Spanish by Nueva Editorial Interamericana S.A., Mexico City, Mexico.

Neurologic Clinics is covered in *Current Contents/Clinical Medicine, MEDLINE/PubMed (Index Medicus), EMBASE/Excerpta Medica,* and *PsycINFO,* and *ISI/BIOMED.*

Contributors

CONSULTING EDITOR

RANDOLPH W. EVANS, MD
Clinical Professor, Department of Neurology, Baylor College of Medicine, Houston, Texas

EDITORS

DAVID E. NEWMAN-TOKER, MD, PhD
Associate Professor of Neurology, Otolaryngology, Emergency Medicine, and Epidemiology, Departments of Neurology, Otolaryngology, and Epidemiology, The Johns Hopkins University School of Medicine & Bloomberg School of Public Health, The Johns Hopkins Hospital, Baltimore, Maryland

KEVIN A. KERBER, MD, MS
Associate Professor of Neurology, Department of Neurology, University of Michigan Health System, Ann Arbor, Michigan

WILLIAM J. MEURER, MD, MS
Assistant Professor, Departments of Emergency Medicine and Neurology, University of Michigan Health System, University of Michigan, Ann Arbor, Michigan

RODNEY OMRON, MD, MPH
Assistant Professor of Emergency Medicine, The Johns Hopkins University School of Medicine, Baltimore, Maryland

JONATHAN A. EDLOW, MD
Professor of Medicine, and Emergency Medicine, Harvard Medical School; Vice Chairman, Department of Emergency Medicine, Beth Israel Deaconess Medical Center, Boston, Massachusetts

AUTHORS

CAREY D. BALABAN, PhD
Departments of Otolaryngology, Neurobiology, Communication Science and Disorders and Bioengineering, Eye and Ear Institute, University of Pittsburgh, Pittsburgh, Pennsylvania

ALEXANDRE R. BISDORFF, MD, PhD
Department of Neurology, Centre Hospitalier Emile Mayrisch, Esch-sur-Alzette, Luxembourg

CHRISTINA A. BLUM, MD
Instructor, Department of Neurology, University of Pennsylvania, Philadelphia, Pennsylvania

ANDREW PHILLIP BRADSHAW, BE, BSc
Institute of Clinical Neurosciences, Royal Prince Alfred Hospital, Central Clinical School, University of Sydney, Sydney, New South Wales, Australia

JONATHAN A. EDLOW, MD
Professor of Medicine, and Emergency Medicine, Harvard Medical School; Vice Chairman, Department of Emergency Medicine, Beth Israel Deaconess Medical Center, Boston, Massachusetts

TERRY D. FIFE, MD
Department of Neurology, Barrow Neurological Institute, University of Arizona College of Medicine, Phoenix, Arizona

GABOR MICHAEL HALMAGYI, MB BS, MD, FRACP
Institute of Clinical Neurosciences, Royal Prince Alfred Hospital, Central Clinical School, University of Sydney, Sydney, New South Wales, Australia

MICHAEL E. HOFFER, MD, FACS
Department of Otolaryngology, University of Miami, Miami, Florida

DIEGO KASKI, MBBS, PhD
Division of Brain Sciences, Charing Cross Hospital, Imperial College London, London, United Kingdom

SCOTT E. KASNER, MD
Professor, Department of Neurology, University of Pennsylvania, Philadelphia, Pennsylvania

KEVIN A. KERBER, MD, MS
Associate Professor of Neurology, Department of Neurology, University of Michigan Health System, Ann Arbor, Michigan

JI-SOO KIM, MD, PhD
Department of Neurology, Seoul National University Bundang Hospital, Seoul National University College of Medicine, Seoul, Korea

CORINNA LECHNER, MPhil
Institute of Clinical Neurosciences, Royal Prince Alfred Hospital, Central Clinical School, University of Sydney, Sydney, New South Wales, Australia

SEUNG-HAN LEE, MD, PhD
Department of Neurology, Chonnam National University Medical School, Gwangju, Korea

JOSE ANTONIO LOPEZ-ESCAMEZ, MD, PhD
Otology and Neurotology Group CTS495, Department of Otolaryngology, Hospital de Poniente, Almería, Spain

PHILLIP A. LOW, MD
Professor, Department of Neurology, Mayo Clinic, Rochester, Minnesota

MANS MAGNUSSON, MD
Professor of Otorhinolaryngology, Department of Otolaryngology, Lund University, Lund, Sweden

WILLIAM J. MEURER, MD, MS
Assistant Professor, Departments of Emergency Medicine and Neurology, University of Michigan Health System, University of Michigan, Ann Arbor, Michigan

DAVID E. NEWMAN-TOKER, MD, PhD
Associate Professor of Neurology, Otolaryngology, Emergency Medicine, and
Epidemiology, Departments of Neurology, Otolaryngology, and Epidemiology,
The Johns Hopkins University School of Medicine & Bloomberg School of Public Health,
The Johns Hopkins Hospital, Baltimore, Maryland

MICHAEL C. SCHUBERT, PT, PhD
Departments of Otolaryngology–Head and Neck Surgery and Physical Medicine and
Rehabilitation, The Johns Hopkins University School of Medicine, Baltimore, Maryland

BARRY SEEMUNGAL, BSc, MB BCh, PhD, FRCP
Division of Brain Sciences, Charing Cross Hospital, Imperial College London, London,
United Kingdom

JEFFREY P. STAAB, MD, MS
Associate Professor, Department of Psychiatry and Psychology, Mayo Clinic, Rochester,
Minnesota

MICHAEL STRUPP, MD, FANA, FEAN
Professor, Department of Neurology, German Center for Vertigo and Balance Disorders,
University Hospital Munich, Munich, Germany

MICHAEL VON BREVERN, MD
Department for Neurology, Park-Klinik Weissensee, Berlin, Germany

MIRIAM S. WELGAMPOLA, MB BS, PhD, FRACP
Institute of Clinical Neurosciences, Royal Prince Alfred Hospital, Central Clinical School,
University of Sydney, Sydney, New South Wales, Australia

Contents

Classifications and definitions are essential to facilitate communication; promote accurate diagnostic criteria; develop, test, and use effective therapies; and specify knowledge gaps. This article describes the development of the International Classification of Vestibular Disorders (ICVD) initiative. It describes its history, scope, and goals. The Bárány Society has played a central role in organizing the ICVD by establishing internal development processes and outreach to other scientific societies. The ICVD is organized in four layers. The current focus is on disorders with a high epidemiologic importance, such as Menière disease, benign paroxysmal positional vertigo, vestibular migraine, and behavioral aspects of vestibular disorders.

 Videos of a left peripheral vestibulopathy; cerebellar nystagmus; the effect of visual fixation on central and peripheral nystagmus; left posterior canal BPV; right horizontal canal BPV; nystagmus simulation created from 2-D video data; paroxysmal torsional downbeat nystagmus; and nystagmus simulation created from 2-D video data accompany this article

Dizziness is a common symptom in emergency departments, general practice, and outpatient clinics. Faced with an acutely dizzy patient, the frontline physician must determine whether or not the symptoms are vestibular in origin and, if they are, which vestibular disorder they best fit. A focused history provides useful clues to the likely cause of dizziness, yet it is the clinical examination that yields the final answer. This article summarizes history and examination techniques that are useful in the assessment of acutely dizzy patients and discusses oculomotor signs that accompany common vestibular disorders.

This article highlights 5 pitfalls in the diagnosis of common vestibular disorders: (1) overreliance on dizziness symptom type to drive diagnostic inquiry; (2) underuse and misuse of timing and triggers to categorize patients; (3) underuse, misuse, and misconceptions linked to hallmark eye examination findings; (4) overweighting age, vascular risk factors, and neurologic examination to screen for stroke; and (5) overuse and overreliance on head computed tomography to rule out neurologic causes. This article discusses the evidence base describing each pitfall's frequency and likely causes, and potential alternative strategies that might be used to improve diagnostic accuracy or mitigate harms.

Diagnosing dizziness can be challenging, and the consequences of missing dangerous causes, such as stroke, can be substantial. Most physicians use a diagnostic paradigm developed more than 40 years ago that focuses on the type of dizziness, but this approach is flawed. This article proposes a new paradigm based on symptom timing, triggers, and targeted bedside eye examinations (TiTrATE). Acute patients fall into 1 of 4 major syndrome categories, each with its own differential diagnosis and set of targeted examination techniques that help make a specific diagnosis. Following an evidence-based approach could help reduce the frequency of misdiagnosis of serious causes of dizziness.

Online Appendix: Acute Dizziness and Vertigo Interactive Case Unknowns
Rodney Omron (with contributions from Sergio Carmona, Joshua N. Goldstein, Jorge C. Kattah, and Sudhir Kothari)

In the spirit of the flipped classroom, the editors of this *Neurologic Clinics* issue on emergency neuro-otology have assembled a collection of unknown cases to be accessed electronically in multimedia format. By design, cases are not linked with specific articles, to avoid untoward cueing effects for the learner. The cases are real and are meant to demonstrate and reinforce lessons provided in this and subsequent articles. In addition to pertinent elements of medical history, cases include videos of key examination findings.

Section II – Acute, Episodic Dizziness and Vertigo

Benign paroxysmal positional vertigo (BPPV) is a common cause of vertigo characterized by brief episodes provoked by head movements. The first attack of BPPV usually occurs in bed or upon getting up. Because it often begins abruptly, it can be alarming and lead to emergency department evaluation. The episodes of spinning often last 10 to 20 seconds, but may occasionally last as long as 1 minute. There are several forms of BPPV. In nearly all cases, highly effective treatment can be offered to patients. This article reviews the current state of our understanding of this condition and its management.

Vestibular migraine is the most common cause of acute episodic vestibular symptoms after benign paroxysmal positional vertigo. In contrast, Ménière's disease is an uncommon disorder. For both conditions, early and accurate diagnosis (or its exclusion) enables the correct management of patients with acute episodic vestibular symptoms. Long-term management of migraine requires changes in lifestyle to avoid triggers of migraine and/or prophylactic drugs if attacks become too frequent. The long-term management of Ménière's disease also involves lifestyle changes (low salt diet), medications (betahistine, steroids), and ablative therapy applied to the diseased ear (eg, intratympanic gentamicin).

Dizziness with or without associated neurologic symptoms is the most common symptom of posterior circulation transient ischemic attack (TIA) and can be more frequent before posterior circulation strokes. This entity carries a high risk of recurrent events and should be considered as a potential cause of spontaneous episodic vestibular syndrome. Diagnostic evaluation should include intracranial and extracranial imaging of the vertebral arteries and basilar artery. Aggressive medical management with antiplatelet therapy, statin use, and risk factor modification is the mainstay of treatment. This article highlights the importance of diagnosing, evaluating, and treating posterior circulation TIAs manifesting as dizziness or vertigo.

Dizziness and vertigo are among the most common presenting patient complaints in ambulatory settings. Specific vestibular causes are often not immediately identifiable. The first task of the clinician is to attempt to rule in specific vestibular disorders, such as benign paroxysmal positional vertigo through physical examination, diagnostic testing, and history taking. A large proportion of patients with dizziness and vertigo will not be easily classified or confirmed as having a specific vestibular cause. As with any undifferentiated patient, the focus in this setting is to attempt to exclude serious or threatening causes.

Mild traumatic brain injury (mTBI) is a common health condition in amateur and professional sports and in military operations but can occur in everyday life. Dizziness is the most common disorder seen after mTBI followed closely by headache. This article examines the diagnosis and treatment of vestibular disorders after mTBI. Data are included from the literature, and conclusions are drawn from the literature review and the experience of the authors. Much of what is known about this disorder comes from recent military experience, but the link to more common civilian injuries is detailed in this article.

 Videos of spontaneous horizontal nystagmus to the right with a very low intensity during fixation; blocking visual fixation with Frenzel's glasses; headimpulse testing; pathological Romberg testing with a fall to the left after closing the eyes; and pathological tandem Romberg with a fall to the left after closing the eyes accompany this article

Normal vestibular end organs generate an equal resting-firing frequency of the axons, which is the same on both sides under static conditions. An acute unilateral vestibulopathy leads to a vestibular tone imbalance. Acute unilateral vestibulopathy is defined by the patient history and the clinical examination and, in unclear cases, laboratory examinations. Key signs and symptoms are an acute onset of spinning vertigo, postural imbalance and nausea as well as a horizontal rotatory nystagmus beating towards the non-affected side, a pathological head-impulse test and no evidence for central vestibular or ocular motor dysfunction. The so-called big five allow a differentiation between a peripheral and central lesion by the bedside examination. The differential diagnosis of peripheral labyrinthine and vestibular nerve disorders mimicking acute unilateral vestibulopathy includes central vestibular disorders, in particular "vestibular pseudoneuritis" and other peripheral vestibular disorders, such as beginning Menière's disease. The management of acute unilateral vestibulopathy involves (1) symptomatic treatment with antivertiginous drugs, (2) causal treatment with corticosteroids, and (3) physical therapy.

Video of head impulse tests accompanies this article

Stroke involving the brainstem and cerebellum frequently presents acute vestibular syndrome. Although vascular vertigo is known to usually accompany other neurologic symptoms and signs, isolated vertigo from small infarcts involving the cerebellum or brainstem has been increasingly recognized. Bedside neuro-otologic examination can reliably differentiate acute vestibular syndrome due to stroke from more benign inner ear disease. Sometimes acute isolated audiovestibular loss may herald impending infarction in the territory of the anterior inferior cerebellar artery. Accurate identification of isolated vascular vertigo is very important because misdiagnosis of acute stroke may result in significant morbidity and mortality.

Most patients with the acute vestibular syndrome (AVS) have vestibular neuritis or stroke or, in the setting of trauma, a posttraumatic vestibular cause. Some medical and nonstroke causes of the AVS must also be considered. Multiple sclerosis is the most common diagnosis in this group. Other less common causes include cerebellar masses, inflammation and infection, mal de debarquement, various toxins, Wernicke disease, celiac-related dizziness, and bilateral vestibulopathy. Finally, there may be unmasking of prior posterior circulation events by various physiologic alterations such as alterations of temperature, blood pressure, electrolytes, or various medications, especially sedating agents.

NEUROLOGIC CLINICS

FORTHCOMING ISSUES

November 2015
Motor Neuron Disease
Richard Barohn and
Mazen Dimachkie, *Editors*

February 2016
**Neurobehavioral Manifestations of
Neurological Diseases: Diagnosis and
Treatment**
Alireza Minagar, Glen Finney, and
Kenneth M. Heilman, *Editors*

May 2016
**Optimal Care for Patients with Epilepsy:
Practical Aspects**
Steven C. Schachter, *Editor*

RECENT ISSUES

May 2015
**Cerebrovascular Diseases: Controversies
and Challenges**
William J. Powers, *Editor*

February 2015
Movement Disorders
Joseph Jankovic, *Editor*

November 2014
Cerebellar Diseases
Alireza Minagar and
Alejandro A. Rabinstein, *Editors*

RELATED INTEREST

Otolaryngologic Clinics of North America, April 2014 (Vol. 47, No. 2)
Headache in Otolaryngology: Rhinogenic and Beyond
Howard Levine and Michael Setzen, *Editors*

THE CLINICS ARE AVAILABLE ONLINE!
Access your subscription at:
www.theclinics.com

Preface

Why Acute Dizziness and Vertigo? Articulating the Emergency Neuro-Otology Imperative

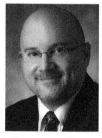
David E. Newman-Toker, MD, PhD

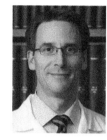
Kevin A. Kerber, MD, MS

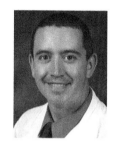
William J. Meurer, MD, MS

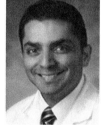
Rodney Omron, MD, MPH

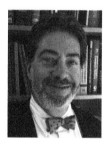
Jonathan A. Edlow, MD

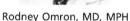
Editors

The focus of this issue is on the patient who presents for urgent or emergent care with a chief complaint of new, previously undiagnosed dizziness or vertigo. Our intended target audience is clinicians from diverse disciplines that evaluate these patients in frontline health care settings. This includes emergency physicians and neurologists, but also otolaryngologists, vestibular physical therapists, and physicians' assistants, among others. Although much of the information presented is

Neurol Clin 33 (2015) xiii–xv
http://dx.doi.org/10.1016/j.ncl.2015.05.001
0733-8619/15/$ – see front matter © 2015 Published by Elsevier Inc.

neurologic.theclinics.com

familiar to subspecialists in neuro-otology or oto-neurology, we hope that our issue offers a comprehensive overview of emergency neuro-otology that has not previously been assembled.

The systematic study of acute dizziness and vertigo in the emergency care setting has grown rapidly over the past decade. Real-world clinical practice has, unfortunately, lagged behind major advances in scientific understanding of vestibular disorders. Many patients with common disorders are still misdiagnosed or mismanaged, with adverse consequences for individual patients (eg, incorrect treatments for common vestibular diseases such as benign paroxysmal positional vertigo and poor outcomes from missed opportunities to treat dangerous strokes presenting acute vertigo). Furthermore, scarce health care resources are being used suboptimally to evaluate these patients.

To help balance between offering state-of-the-art vestibular science and accessibility for the general reader, I have deliberately engaged emergency physician coeditors and authors who bring an expert frontline provider perspective. I have chosen four coeditors, each of whom has made important contributions to the study and teaching of vestibular diagnosis or management in the acute care setting. Kevin Kerber is a vestibular neurologist known for his health services research in acute dizziness, including several key studies focused on the delivery of emergency care for benign positional vertigo and stroke. Our three other coeditors are experienced emergency physicians who bring a true, card-carrying emergency medicine perspective to this acute-care–focused issue. Will Meurer brings a rigorous research methods background to the study of emergency neurology and also years of bedside research on the topic of dizziness. Rodney Omron brings a strong background in curriculum development and educational innovation for vertigo. Jonathan Edlow brings the experience of a seasoned clinician and educator known in the United States and internationally as the leading emergency medicine practitioner and teacher on dizziness and vertigo.

We hope to emphasize throughout the issue five primary components of initial diagnosis and management:

1. Epidemiology, differential diagnosis, and disease definitions;
2. Bedside clinical features that differentiate dangerous from benign causes;
3. Appropriate use of advanced diagnostic tests (including imaging, vestibular tests) and consultations;
4. Application of early treatments (manipulative, pharmacologic, rehabilitative);
5. Acute disposition strategies, including determining need for admission and urgency of follow-up.

The issue is divided into three major sections devoted to (1) overall approach to initial diagnosis and management (with interactive cases included as an additional online resource for self-study), (2) specific disorders causing episodic symptoms, and (3) specific disorders causing acute, continuous symptoms. This issue structure is designed to emphasize the typical approach that would be applied using best-evidence–based clinical practice, which differs critically between patients with episodic symptoms and those with acute, continuous symptoms.

We have tried to discuss topics and content in proportion to clinical relevance of these disorders in the acute care setting (rather than their relevance to vestibular specialists per se). Accordingly, we have, in places, combined disease topics traditionally treated separately. Again, this choice is deliberate, since it reinforces for the reader the conceptual similarity in diagnosis and initial management for disorders that may present with similar early phenotypes or be managed similarly during the acute phase (eg, vestibular migraine and Menière disease).

We hope that our fresh perspective and synthesis of recent advances offers both generalist and specialist clinicians a resource to provide the highest-quality, evidence-based care for their patients with acute dizziness and vertigo.

David E. Newman-Toker, MD, PhD
Johns Hopkins Hospital
CRB-II, Room 2M-03 North
1550 Orleans Street
Baltimore, MD 21231, USA

Kevin A. Kerber, MD, MS
Department of Neurology
University of Michigan Health System
1500 East Medical Center Drive
Ann Arbor, MI 48109, USA

William J. Meurer, MD, MS
University of Michigan
TC B1-354/5303
1500 East Medical Center Drive
Ann Arbor, MI 48109, USA

Rodney Omron, MD, MPH
The Johns Hopkins University School of Medicine
1830 East Monument Street, Suite 6-100
Baltimore, MD 21287, USA

Jonathan A. Edlow, MD
Department of Emergency Medicine
Beth Israel Deaconess Medical Center
Administrative Offices
West CC-2
1 Deaconess Place
Boston, MA 02215, USA

E-mail addresses:
toker@jhu.edu (D.E. Newman-Toker)
kakerber@med.umich.edu (K.A. Kerber)
wmeurer@med.umich.edu (W.J. Meurer)
romron1@jhmi.edu (R. Omron)
jedlow@bidmc.harvard.edu (J.A. Edlow)

Section I – Overall Approach to Acute Dizziness and Vertigo

Overview of the International Classification of Vestibular Disorders

Alexandre R. Bisdorff, MD, PhD[a],*, Jeffrey P. Staab, MD, MS[b],
David E. Newman-Toker, MD, PhD[c]

KEYWORDS

- Vestibular • Vertigo • Symptoms • Classification • Bárány Society

KEY POINTS

- Classifications and definitions are essential to facilitate communication between clinicians and researchers and promote diagnostic criteria and research in mechanisms epidemiology and treatment.
- To build the International Classification of Vestibular Disorders (ICVD), the Bárány Society organized a systematic internal process and processes for encouraging consensus with other scientific societies.
- The ICVD is organized in 4 layers: (1) symptoms and signs, (2) syndromes, (3) disorders and diseases, and (4) mechanisms.
- Definitions for vestibular symptoms and vestibular migraine have been published. Those for benign paroxysmal positional vertigo, Menière disease, and behavioral aspects should follow in 2015.

INTRODUCTION

Symptom and disease definitions are a fundamental prerequisite for professional communication in clinical, research, and public health settings. The need for structured criteria for epidemiologic, diagnostic and therapeutic research is more obvious for disciplines that rely heavily on syndromic diagnosis, such as psychiatry and headache, where there are currently no histopathologic, radiographic, physiologic, or other confirmatory diagnostic tests available. However, diagnostic standards and

[a] Department of Neurology, Centre Hospitalier Emile Mayrisch, rue Emile Mayrisch, Esch-sur-Alzette 4005, Luxembourg; [b] Department of Psychiatry and Psychology, Mayo Clinic, 200 1st Street SW, Rochester, MN 55905, USA; [c] Departments of Neurology, Otolaryngology, and Epidemiology, The Johns Hopkins University School of Medicine & Bloomberg School of Public Health, The Johns Hopkins Hospital, CRB-II, Room 2M-03 North, 1550 Orleans Street, Baltimore, MD 21231, USA
* Corresponding author.
E-mail address: alexbis@pt.lu

Neurol Clin 33 (2015) 541–550
http://dx.doi.org/10.1016/j.ncl.2015.04.010
neurologic.theclinics.com
0733-8619/15/$ – see front matter © 2015 Elsevier Inc. All rights reserved.

classifications are also crucial in areas of medicine, such as epilepsy and rheumatology, where, although confirmatory tests do exist, there is substantial overlap in clinical features or biomarkers across syndromes. Vestibular disorders are similar to the latter examples. Scientific and therapeutic progress, as well as public awareness of psychiatric and headache disorders, vastly increased after the introduction of the first modern version of the Diagnostic and Statistical Manual of Mental Disorders (DSM-III) by the American Psychiatric Association in 1980[1] and the first International Classification of Headache Disorders by the International Headache Society in 1988.[2]

Although numerous advances in basic and clinical vestibular research have been made, progress in the field likely has been hampered by the lack of explicit and uniform criteria for the description of symptoms, syndromes, and clinical disorders. Other than the definition of Menière disease by the Japanese Society for Equilibrium Research and the American Academy of Otolaryngology—Head and Neck Surgery[3] as well as the Classification of Peripheral Vestibular Disorders by the Spanish Society of Otorhinolaryngology,[4] there have not been systematic efforts to create widely accepted classification criteria before the initiative by the Bárány Society to build the International Classification of Vestibular Disorders (ICVD).[5]

There are probably several reasons why the classification and unification of definitions for vestibular disorders has lagged other illnesses. Classifications are usually created by scientific societies of subspecialists within a medical specialty or under the lead of 1 medical specialty. Vestibular disorders cross medical specialist boundaries and, despite being very prevalent,[6] are the province of small subspecialties within otolaryngology and neurology. Additionally, for neurologists and otolaryngologists to be able to cover competently the spectrum of differential diagnoses of vestibular disorders, they need to acquire elaborate knowledge about the inner ear, vestibular, postural, and oculomotor pathways in the brain, and related systems that control autonomic and threat responses, which goes beyond the standard curricula during residency training of any specialty. It was, therefore, necessary that an international scientific society with an interdisciplinary membership of clinicians and basic scientists with expertise in vestibular disorders, like the Bárány Society,[7] assume responsibility for developing the ICVD.

GOALS AND SCOPE FOR THE INTERNATIONAL CLASSIFICATION OF VESTIBULAR DISORDERS INITIATIVE

The goal of the ICVD initiative is to develop a comprehensive classification scheme and definitions of individual vestibular diseases disorders that is acceptable worldwide. To achieve the goal of wide acceptance, the Bárány Society is actively seeking the input of members from other associations dealing with vestibular disorders, such as the Société Internationale d'Otoneurologie and the Comisión de Otoneurología de la Sociedad Española de Otorrinolaringología in Europe, the American Academy of Otolaryngology – Head and Neck Surgery (AAO-HNS) in the United States, the Japanese Equilibrium Society, and the Korean Balance Society, as well as individual scientists and clinicians from the international vestibular community. Beyond cooperation with individuals and associations within the vestibular community, the Bárány Society is also seeking cooperation and consensus with scientific associations from related disciplines, if there are important aspects of diseases that touch more than 1 society. One example is vestibular migraine, where the Bárány Society cooperated with the International Headache Society to publish a consensus document on diagnostic criteria.[8]

The term "vestibular disorders" refers to disturbances arising from the vestibular system, but the definition of the vestibular system itself can be understood broadly or narrowly. The vestibular system contributes to gait, stance, locomotion, balance, vision, spatial orientation, navigation, and spatial memory because of the widespread use of vestibular information in the brain. Furthermore, brain dysfunction of almost any cause, whether primary or secondary, may affect balance adversely. It is therefore necessary to limit the scope of problems classified as "vestibular disorders" within the ICVD, although some decisions will ultimately be arbitrary.

The ICVD will include diseases that affect the vestibular labyrinth of the inner ear, connections from the labyrinth to the brain at the brainstem, the cerebellum, subcortical structures that process spatial stimuli, and the vestibular cortex. The ICVD will also include illnesses that are primarily the province of other specialties, but produce symptoms that mimic vestibular disorders. The ICVD will focus on the vestibular presentations of these conditions, but will not seek to redefine or reclassify the primary nonvestibular disorder. Examples include syncope, seizures, stroke, headache disorders, cerebellar ataxia syndromes, extrapyramidal movement disorders, and behavioral disorders that are already defined by other groups. The classification will eventually include controversial and emerging entities, such as cervical vertigo,[9] in the hope that identifying limits of current scientific knowledge will prompt research to fill these gaps.

Before starting the task of elaborating definitions of disorders the problem of variable use of terminology for describing core vestibular symptoms, such as dizziness and vertigo, had to be addressed. Even when studied in a single, English-speaking country, the term "vertigo" has been shown to have diverse meanings for patients,[10] generalist physicians,[11] and even otologists.[12]

METHODOLOGY AND PROCESS FOR DEVELOPING THE INTERNATIONAL CLASSIFICATION OF VESTIBULAR DISORDERS

In 2006 the Classification Committee of the Bárány Society (CCBS) convened its first meeting to begin structuring the approach to developing the ICVD. The group needed to develop a conceptual framework, a list of initial topics, and a process for consensus building. To permit terminological consistency in defining vestibular disorders as part of the ICVD, it was decided to first define key vestibular symptoms and build consensus around these formalized definitions (**Boxes 1** and **2**); the product of this initial work has already been published.[5] Initial topics (eg, Menière disease, vestibular migraine, benign paroxysmal positional vertigo) were chosen for their frequency and importance to the vestibular disorders community. Specific issues are delegated to subcommittees working according to predetermined guidelines. Subcommittees

---

Box 1
Glossary of primary vestibular symptom definitions in the International Classification of Vestibular Disorders

Dizziness is the sensation of disturbed or impaired spatial orientation without a false or distorted sense of motion.

Vertigo is the sensation of self-motion (of head/body) when no self-motion is occurring or the sensation of distorted self-motion during an otherwise normal head movement.

Vestibulovisual symptoms are visual symptoms that usually result from vestibular pathology or the interplay between visual and vestibular systems. These include false sensations of motion or tilting of the visual surround and visual distortion (blur) linked to vestibular (rather than optical) failure.

Postural symptoms are balance symptoms related to maintenance of postural stability, occurring only while upright (seated, standing, or walking).

Box 2
Glossary of secondary vestibular symptom definitions in the International Classification of Vestibular Disorders

Spontaneous vertigo (or dizziness) is vertigo (or dizziness) that occurs without an obvious trigger.

Triggered vertigo (or dizziness) is vertigo (or dizziness) that occurs with an obvious trigger.

- *Positional vertigo (or dizziness)* is vertigo (or dizziness) triggered by and occurring *after* a change of head position in space relative to gravity.

- *Head motion vertigo (or dizziness)* is vertigo (or dizziness) occurring only *during* head motion (ie, that is time locked to the head movement).

- *Visually induced vertigo (or dizziness)* is vertigo (or dizziness) triggered by a complex, distorted, large field, or moving visual stimulus, including the relative motion of the visual surround associated with body movement.

- *Sound-induced vertigo (or dizziness)* is vertigo (or dizziness) triggered by an auditory stimulus.

- *Valsalva-induced vertigo (or dizziness)* is vertigo (or dizziness) triggered by any bodily maneuver that tends to increase intracranial or middle ear pressure.

- *Orthostatic vertigo (or dizziness)* is vertigo (or dizziness) triggered by and occurring on arising (ie, a change of body posture from lying to sitting or sitting to standing).

Vestibulovisual symptoms

- *External vertigo* is the false sensation that the visual surround is spinning or flowing.

- *Oscillopsia* is the false sensation that the visual surround is oscillating.

- *Visual lag* is the false sensation that the visual surround follows behind a head movement with a delay or makes a brief drift after the head movement is completed.

- *Visual tilt* is the false perception of the visual surround as oriented off the true vertical.

- *Movement-induced blur* is reduced visual acuity during or momentarily after a head movement.

Postural symptoms

- *Unsteadiness* is the feeling of being unstable while seated, standing, or walking without a particular directional preference.

- *Directional pulsion* is the feeling of being unstable with a tendency to veer or fall in a particular direction while seated, standing, or walking. The direction should be specified as latero-, retro-, or anteropulsion. If lateropulsion, the direction (right or left) should be specified.

- A *balance-related near fall* is a sensation of imminent fall (without a completed fall) related to strong unsteadiness, directional pulsion, or other vestibular symptom (eg, vertigo).

- A *balance-related fall* is a completed fall related to strong unsteadiness, directional pulsion, or other vestibular symptom (eg, vertigo).

---

have a designated chair, who is a member of the Bárány Society. He or she composes his or her subcommittee, which must include members from 3 continents, at least 1 clinician must be an otolaryngologist and 1 a neurologist. Clinicians and scientists from other fields are included, based on needs for additional expertise.

The work of a subcommittee is part of a consensus process based on the best available evidence at present. Each subcommittee's work is subject to review by the CCBS. Draft definitions are presented publically at the biennial Bárány Society congresses and posted online for a period of commentary by Bárány Society members. Input is also solicited from other scientific societies based on the topic treated. The CCBS oversees the whole process to ensure that all the parts of the classification are coherent with each other. The final document is then published in the *Journal of Vestibular Research* without further peer review and is then available as open access publication.

INTERNATIONAL CLASSIFICATION OF VESTIBULAR DISORDERS STRUCTURE

The proposed structure of the ICVD currently includes 4 layers. Layer I, symptoms and signs; layer II, clinical syndromes; layer III-A, diseases and disorders; and layer III-B, pathophysiologic mechanisms (**Fig. 1**). Each layer contains elements (eg, specific symptoms or diseases) that are important in their own right, but are also important in their links with other elements. This structure will allow the ICVD to depict conceptual connections between elements within and across layers. Because knowledge of these connections is incomplete, it is recognized that some links may also "skip" layers.

A multilayer approach was considered essential to accommodate the breadth of clinical and research applications, now and in the future. Some clinicians and researchers must organize their approach beginning with signs and symptoms, whereas others must lead with a primary focus on specific diseases or pathophysiologic mechanisms.

INTERNATIONAL CLASSIFICATION OF VESTIBULAR DISORDERS LAYER I: SYMPTOMS AND SIGNS

Definitions for specific vestibular symptoms in layer I of the ICVD have been written and published.[5] Work is underway on specific signs, particularly pathologic eye

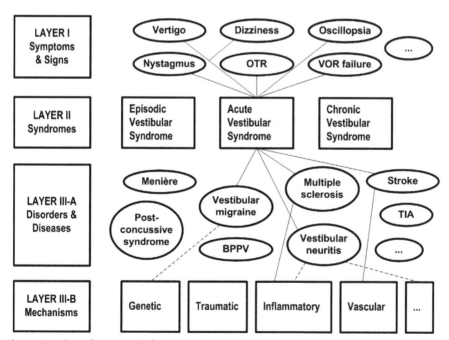

Fig. 1. Four-layer framework of the international classification of vestibular disorders. Links between layers are shown demonstrating, in this case, the conceptual relations between the "acute vestibular syndrome" (layer II), its component symptoms (layer I), its etiologic causes (layer III-A), and their mechanistic underpinnings (layer III-B). Solid lines represent definite links, and dashed lines represent uncertain links. OTR, ocular tilt reaction; TIA, transient ischemic attack.

movements. This layer was addressed first because it was considered foundational to the development of all subsequent definitions, the vast majority of which will be based on clinical phenomena. It was decided to limit the scope of this work to defining cardinal vestibular symptoms, representing the primary clinical symptoms typically resulting from vestibular disorders but excluding secondary symptoms such as nausea, fatigue, and anxiety.

The principles followed for developing symptom definitions were as follows:

- No "vestibular" symptom has a totally specific meaning in terms of topology or nosology and its pathogenesis is likely to be incompletely understood.
- Symptom definitions should be as purely phenomenological as possible, without reference to a specific theory on pathophysiologic causes of a particular disease.
- Definitions for symptoms are clearest if they are nonoverlapping and nonhierarchical, allowing for 1 or more symptoms to coexist in a particular patient.

The ICVD describes 4 categories of cardinal vestibular symptoms: (1) vertigo, (2) dizziness, (3) vestibulovisual symptoms, and (4) postural symptoms, including subtypes for each.[5] The new nomenclature distinguishes *vertigo* (a false sense of motion of spinning or nonspinning quality) and *dizziness* (disturbed spatial orientation without a false sense of motion), which represents an important departure from typical practice in the United States, where dizziness is an umbrella term encompassing vertigo, unsteadiness, imbalance, presyncope, and other 'nonspecific' sensations.[11] Although vertigo and dizziness are distinguished from one another in the ICVD, neither is considered pathognomonic in its links to underlying vestibular pathology. Both symptoms are frequently encountered in patients with vestibular or nonvestibular disorders, whether acute or chronic.[10,13] Vertigo and dizziness are each divided into 2 categories, spontaneous and triggered.

A separate category on vestibulovisual symptoms was developed, because vestibular dysfunction can result in a range of visual disturbances. Because "internal" and "external" vertigo are sometimes dissociated clinically (eg, in a patient who sees the world spinning or rotating from jerk nystagmus, but feels no spinning with eyes closed), the visual sense of motion could not simply be incorporated into the definition of vertigo. The term "external vertigo," referring to false sensations of motion in the visual surround, was listed among the vestibulovisual symptoms. Although some prior studies[6] have called this sense of visual flux "oscillopsia," group consensus was that oscillopsia should be restricted to describing a bidirectional, oscillating visual motion that incorporates complaints such as "jumping" or "bouncing" vision.

The ICVD definitions for postural balance symptoms use *unsteadiness* as the preferred descriptive term for postural instability when upright (ie, sensations of swaying, rocking, or wobbling when sitting, standing, or walking), rather than the more linguistically ambiguous terms "disequilibrium" or "imbalance." If the unsteadiness has a particular directional bias, the term *directional pulsion* should be used and the direction specified (eg, lateropulsion to the right). A subcommittee devoted to signs is currently establishing a classification and definitions of various forms of nystagmus.

INTERNATIONAL CLASSIFICATION OF VESTIBULAR DISORDERS LAYER II: SYNDROMES

Layer II, syndromes, offers an intermediate layer of syndromic classification that bridges between constellations of symptoms and signs and the diseases or disorders causing them. For example, sudden-onset vertigo, nausea, vomiting, head motion intolerance, gait unsteadiness, and nystagmus would constitutive an "acute vestibular syndrome" that has underlying causes, such as vestibular neuritis and acute cerebellar infarction. Currently proposed are 3 specific syndromes comprising the bulk of all vestibular presentations: (1) acute vestibular syndrome comprising diseases and disorders that usually manifest with a single episode of sudden onset vestibular symptoms and signs (eg, vestibular neuritis or acute stroke), (2) episodic vestibular syndrome comprising diseases and disorders that are recurrent by nature (eg, Menière disease, vestibular migraine, or transient ischemic attack), and (3) chronic vestibular syndrome comprising diseases and disorders that produce persistent vestibular symptoms and signs over an extended period of time (bilateral vestibular failure or cerebellar degeneration). Layer II will facilitate the development of clinical care pathways and standardized inclusion criteria for research studies focused on diagnostic accuracy.

INTERNATIONAL CLASSIFICATION OF VESTIBULAR DISORDERS LAYER III: DISORDERS AND DISEASES

Layer III-A contains vestibular diseases and disorders and seeks to be relatively comprehensive. The ICVD will use existing terms for vestibular disorders and diseases wherever possible. New terms will be developed only for conditions not included in previous classifications or, rarely, for conditions having multiple names that are all incompatible with ICVD nomenclature. If several existing names are used to describe the same condition, the CCBS will endeavor to include the most suitable one in the ICVD classification system. Other terms will be designated as "terms not used in this nomenclature."

For most vestibular diseases and disorders, no single pathognomonic finding or definitive set of confirmatory tests are available. Therefore, the definitions use operational criteria for symptom dimensions (eg, type, timing, or triggers) or symptom clusters and ancillary test results, as appropriate. Both supporting and negating criteria will be considered. Criteria will be graded to define a range of certainty about a particular diagnosis from *definite* (clear and certain) to *probable* (less clear and less certain). The former will be more restrictive (ie, more specific), whereas the latter will be more inclusive (ie, more sensitive). Denoting a degree of diagnostic certainty is important for both clinical care and research. For example, clinicians will likely apply a high-risk therapy (eg, vestibular neurectomy) only to patients with "definite" disease, although they may be willing to apply a low-risk therapy (eg, dietary modification) to a patient with probable or even "possible" disease.

The CCBS established the first 4 disease-oriented subcommittees to address the definitions and diagnostic criteria for diseases where consensus is most urgently needed because of their epidemiologic importance or ongoing controversy. These subcommittees are focused on Menière disease, benign paroxysmal positional vertigo, vestibular migraine, and behavioral neuro-otologic conditions. The diagnostic criteria for vestibular migraine were the first to be published.[8] The definition of vestibular migraine identifies this condition as a subcategory of migraine, similar to retinal migraine, with vestibular symptoms as a predominant sensory manifestation. The criteria are based on definitions first proposed by Neuhauser and colleagues[14] in 2001 and later formalized by Furman and colleagues.[15,16] The Menière Subcommittee built on the AAO-HNS definition of Menière disease, which has been used worldwide since its publication in 1995.[3] The new definition will only include 2 categories of certainty (definite and probable) and will be more precise regarding hearing loss and the diagnostic overlap with other conditions presenting the episodic vestibular syndrome, mainly vestibular migraine. The Benign Paroxysmal Positional Vertigo Subcommittee prepared detailed definitions of symptoms and signs for all variants of canalolithiasis and cupulolithiasis currently described in the medical literature, subdividing them into established and emerging entities according to available evidence. These definitions are expected to be published in 2015.

The Behavioral Subcommittee was the last of the current working groups to be formed and met for the first time in August 2010 in Reykjavik during the 26th Bárány Society meeting. That subcommittee was charged with 2 tasks: (1) to identify the primary and secondary psychiatric disorders that manifest vestibular symptoms and modify their standard definitions for ease of use by otologists and neuro-otologists, and (2) to evaluate the available data on phobic postural vertigo, chronic subjective dizziness, space–motion discomfort, and visually induced dizziness (previously visual vertigo) to determine whether these entities represent 1 or more disorders, and then prepare a suitable definition or definitions for the ICVD. This task was complicated by the fact that both sets of standardized psychiatric nomenclature were in the process of revision when the subcommittee was formed. The updated version of the DSM (DSM-5) was published in 2013 after a lengthy revision cycle [17]. Its definitions align better with those of the 11th edition of the International Classifications of Diseases (ICD-11),[18] which is still in beta draft version awaiting finalization in 2017. The subcommittee prepared modified definitions of anxiety and depressive disorders that manifest vestibular symptoms for use in neuro-otologic clinical and research settings. It also determined that phobic postural vertigo and chronic subjective dizziness were different descriptions of a single clinical entity with space–motion discomfort and visually induced dizziness as important symptoms. Therefore, the subcommittee defined 1 chronic vestibular syndrome that captures key features of this condition and termed it persistent postural–perceptual dizziness in keeping with ICVD nomenclature. The definition of persistent postural–perceptual dizziness will be posted to the Internet for commentary in spring 2015, with the remaining behavioral vestibular disorders to follow.

INTERNATIONAL CLASSIFICATION OF VESTIBULAR DISORDERS LAYER III-B: MECHANISMS

Layer III-B contains the pathoanatomic, pathophysiologic, and etiologic mechanisms underlying vestibular disorders. It is anticipated that this layer will be developed last and will be the most incomplete in the first iteration of the ICVD, but will expand and grow the most with future scientific discovery. This layer has been created with the knowledge that, eventually, clinical phenomena (ie, symptoms and signs) may be linked directly with mechanistic understanding (eg, genetic mutation) for the purposes of diagnosis and treatment, skipping intermediate steps in the diagnostic process that are unavoidable at present (eg, "diagnosis" of Menière disease).

INTERNATIONAL CLASSIFICATION OF VESTIBULAR DISORDERS AND FUNCTIONAL OUTCOMES

Finally, it is recognized that the functional impact of vestibular diseases and disorders is substantial and that a schema for standardized assessment of disability or handicap is needed. A diagnosis itself does not provide information about functional consequences for the affected individual. The World Health Organization has created the International Classification of Functioning, Disability and Health, which describes the adverse effect of disease on daily activities and makes the assessment of functional impairment and disability caused by diseases of all types systematic and comparable. A working group is developing an instrument to use International Classification of Functioning, Disability and Health measures to assess function in patients with vestibular disorders.

SUMMARY

An initiative under the aegis of the CCBS is currently underway to develop a comprehensive classification structure and formal definitions for vestibular symptoms, syndromes, and diseases. The success of the ICVD will depend on its ability to improve communication among scientists, clinicians, patients, policymakers, and the general public, to advance knowledge about vestibular disorders, and to reduce the morbidity of those afflicted by the conditions it defines.

ACKNOWLEDGMENT

Dr Newman-Toker's effort was supported, in part, by a grant from the National Institutes of Health, National Institute on Deafness and Other Communication Disorders (1U01DC013778-01A1).

REFERENCES

1. American Psychiatric Association. Diagnostic and statistical manual of mental disorders. 3rd edition. Washington, DC: American Psychiatric Association; 1980.
2. Classification and diagnostic criteria for headache disorders, cranial neuralgias and facial pain. Headache Classification Committee of the International Headache Society. Cephalalgia 1988;8(Suppl 7):1–96.
3. Committee on Hearing and Equilibrium guidelines for the diagnosis and evaluation of therapy in Meniere's disease. American Academy of Otolaryngology-Head and Neck Foundation, Inc. Otolaryngol Head Neck Surg 1995;113:181–5.
4. Morera C, Pérez H, Pérez N, et al. Peripheral vertigo classification. Consensus document. Otoneurology Committee of the Spanish Otorhinolaryngology Society (2003-2006). Acta Otorrinolaringol Esp 2008;59(2):76–9.
5. Bisdorff A, von Brevern M, Lempert T, et al. Classification of vestibular symptoms: towards an international classification of vestibular disorders. J Vestib Res 2009; 19(1–2):1–13.
6. Neuhauser H, von Brevern M, Radtke A, et al. Epidemiology of vestibular vertigo: a neurotologic survey of the general population. Neurology 2005;65(6):898–904 [Erratum appears in Neurology 2006;67(8):1528].
7. Bárány Society, The International Society for Neuro-Otology. Available at: www.baranysociety.nl. Accessed January, 2015.
8. Lempert T, Olesen J, Furman J, et al. Vestibular migraine: diagnostic criteria. J Vestib Res 2012;22(4):167–72.
9. Brandt T, Bronstein AM. Nosological entities? Cervical vertigo. J Neurol Neurosurg Psychiatry 2001;71:8–12.
10. Newman-Toker DE, Cannon LM, Stofferahn ME, et al. Imprecision in patient reports of dizziness symptom quality: a cross-sectional study conducted in an acute-care setting. Mayo Clin Proc 2007;82(11):1329–40.
11. Stanton VA, Hsieh YH, Camargo CA Jr, et al. Overreliance on symptom quality in diagnosing dizziness: results of a multicenter survey of emergency physicians. Mayo Clin Proc 2007;82(11):1319–28. [Erratum appears in Mayo Clin Proc 2013;88(7):777].
12. Blakley BW, Goebel J. The meaning of the word "vertigo". Otolaryngol Head Neck Surg 2001;125(3):147–50.
13. Newman-Toker DE, Dy FJ, Stanton VA, et al. How often is dizziness from primary cardiovascular disease true vertigo? A systematic review. J Gen Intern Med 2008; 23(12):2087–94.

14. Neuhauser H, Leopold M, von Brevern M, et al. The interrelations of migraine, vertigo, and migrainous vertigo. Neurology 2001;56:436–41.
15. Furman J, Marcus DA, Balaban CD. Migrainous vertigo: development of a pathogenetic model and structured diagnostic interview. Curr Opin Neurol 2003; 16(1):5–13.
16. Grill E, Furman JM, Alghwiri AA, et al. Using core sets of the international classification of functioning, disability and health (ICF) to measure disability in vestibular disorders: study protocol. J Vestib Res 2013;23(6):297–303.
17. American Psychiatric Association. Diagnostic and Statistical Manual of Mental Disorders, DSM-5. Washington, DC: American Psychiatric Association; 2013.
18. World Health Organization, International Classification of Diseases, 11th edition, beta draft version. Available at: http://apps.who.int/classifications/icd11/browse. Accessed January, 2015.

Bedside Assessment of Acute Dizziness and Vertigo

Miriam S. Welgampola, MB BS, PhD, FRACP*, Andrew Phillip Bradshaw, BE, BSc, Corinna Lechner, MPhil, Gabor Michael Halmagyi, MB BS, MD, FRACP

KEYWORDS

- Nystagmus • Vestibular neuritis • BPV • Meniere disease • Vestibular migraine

KEY POINTS

- Acute vertigo is accompanied by nystagmus that points to its underlying cause. A focused history and careful bedside examination (with emphasis on spontaneous and positional nystagmus characteristics and head impulse testing) yield the underlying diagnosis.
- An acute vestibular syndrome is a sudden severe and prolonged episode of vertigo that could be caused by vestibular neuritis or a stroke. Typical vestibular neuritis is characterized by peripheral nystagmus, a positive bedside head impulse test, absence of skew deviation, and normal hearing. If all 4 conditions are not met, a stroke should be considered.
- Recurrent positional dizziness is most often due to benign positional vertigo (BPV), which is characterized by exclusively positional, paroxysmal vertigo and nystagmus in the plane of the affected semicircular canal.
- Recurrent spontaneous vertigo lasting hours could be due to vestibular migraine, often accompanied by spontaneous horizontal, vertical, or torsional nystagmus, or by Meniere disease, which typically begins with ipsiversive horizontal nystagmus and later progresses to contraversive paretic nystagmus.
- Assessment of an acutely dizzy patient without a means of removing visual fixation is unrewarding, because spontaneous nystagmus is often missed.

Videos of a left peripheral vestibulopathy; cerebellar nystagmus; the effect of visual fixation on central and peripheral nystagmus; left posterior canal BPV; right horizontal canal BPV; nystagmus simulation created from 2-D video data; paroxysmal torsional downbeat nystagmus; and nystagmus simulation created from 2-D video data accompany this article at http://www.neurologic. theclinics.com/

M.S. Welgampola's and G.M. Halmagyi's research is funded by the National Health and Medical Research Council, Australia. A.P. Bradshaw and C. Lechner have nothing to declare.
Institute of Clinical Neurosciences, Royal Prince Alfred Hospital, Central Clinical School, University of Sydney, Sydney, New South Wales, Australia
* Corresponding author.
E-mail address: miriam@icn.usyd.edu.au

Neurol Clin 33 (2015) 551–564
http://dx.doi.org/10.1016/j.ncl.2015.04.001   neurologic.theclinics.com

INTRODUCTION

Acute vertigo is equally unpleasant and anxiety provoking for frontline physicians and patients. Many physicians assessing a dizzy patient fear they might miss a life-threatening brainstem stroke, perform a brain CT that almost never yields useful information to exclude a central cause, administer antiemetics or vestibular suppressants, and discharge a patient from care without a clear diagnosis or treatment. During the past 150 years, the common causes of acute vertigo have been well characterized. With a focused history and careful physical examination, it is now possible correctly diagnose a majority of these disorders and offer useful treatment to patients presenting with acute vertigo. What questions must a clinician ask to determine the cause of vertigo? What might the physical examination reveal? What additional resources could help confirm the diagnosis? This review presents the essential history and bedside examination that can and should be performed in emergency departments, general practice, and outpatient clinics.

THE HISTORY

A focused history is a valuable contributor to a correct diagnosis. Sometimes a patient's opening sentence might provide the diagnosis. "I spin whenever I turn over to one side in bed" is an unmistakable history of BPV. When the open-ended history does not yield the diagnosis, the following key questions need to be addressed.

Is It Truly Vertigo?

Vestibular vertigo is an illusion of movement (spinning, rocking, or tilting) of oneself or one's surroundings and implies a left-right asymmetry in the neural activity of the vestibular nuclei. Light-headedness, fuzzy head, and presyncopal sensations are more commonly reported in nonvestibular dizziness. In an ideal world, the quality of dizziness should help separate vestibular from nonvestibular dizziness (postural hypotension, cardiac rhythm disturbances, syncope, anemia, hypoglycemia, hypercalcemia, vitamin B_{12} deficiency, medication effects, and anxiety). Yet, patients' descriptions are notoriously unreliable; therefore, it is best not to rely entirely on the reported quality of dizziness.[1]

Is It the First Ever Attack or Is It Long-standing Recurrent Vertigo?

The first ever attack of acute spontaneous vertigo lasting 24 hours or longer (also called an acute vestibular syndrome) is most commonly due to vestibular neuritis, which is a benign and self-limiting disorder; however, it could also be due to a cerebellar infarct, which is potentially life threatening. To separate these 2 different entities with a near-identical history, it is essential to learn to elicit the clinical signs of vestibular neuritis.[2,3] Episodic vertigo occurring over many years is harmless in origin and could represent BPV, vestibular migraine, Meniere disease, or vestibular paroxysmia. A recent history of recurrent episodes of vertigo, especially crescendo vertigo (episodes occurring with an increasing severity and frequency) lasting minutes, should ring alarm bells for posterior circulation transient ischemic attacks (TIAs).

Is It Spontaneous or Positional?

All types of vertigo worsen with head movement. Vertigo that is present at rest and worse with any head movement does not constitute positional vertigo. Vertigo that is absent at rest and is brought on only by lying down, turning over in bed, bending down, or arching back is likely to represent BPV. Less commonly, vestibular migraine and vestibular paroxysmia could also present with positional vertigo.[4,5] Postural hypotension can be triggered by arising from the supine or sitting to the upright position. Spontaneous vertigo could be due to vestibular migraine, Meniere disease, vestibular neuritis, and posterior circulation ischemia.

What Is the Duration of Each Spell?

Vertigo lasting only seconds is most commonly due to BPV but also could be due to vestibular migraine or vestibular paroxysmia. Episodes lasting minutes raise the possibility of posterior circulation TIAs or vestibular migraine. Symptoms lasting hours could be due to Meniere disease or vestibular migraine whereas a duration of 24 hours or longer (also called an acute vestibular syndrome) is encountered in vestibular neuritis, stroke, or vestibular migraine.

What Are the Associated Symptoms?

Conventional teaching has been that associated aural symptoms automatically imply peripheral vertigo. Nothing could be further from the truth. Acute unilateral tinnitus and hearing loss in the context of an acute vestibular syndrome could mean an anterior inferior cerebellar artery (AICA) infarction.[6] Aural fullness, tinnitus, and fluctuating hearing loss that herald or accompany vertigo lasting hours are indicative of Meniere disease.[7]

Vertigo associated with migraine headaches, photophobia, phonophobia, or visual aura and a history of profound motion sensitivity make vestibular migraine more likely.[4] Vertigo from brainstem infarction or demyelination can present with associated neurologic symptoms of diplopia, facial paresthesia or weakness, dysarthria, dysphonia or hiccups, limb weakness, clumsiness, or sensory loss. Dizziness associated with panic symptoms triggered by specific situations (supermarkets or crowded public places) could point to anxiety as an underlying cause. Undiagnosed and untreated vestibular vertigo, however, could also lead to subsequent anxiety symptoms that take the foreground.

Do Recent Events Provide a Clue?

If there has been a recent head trauma, consider BPV, skull base fracture with vestibular loss, perilymph fistula, and migraine.[8] A recent introduction of or change in blood pressure–lowering medication might imply postural hypotension. A recent salt load from festive dining might imply the first episode of Meniere disease.

THE PHYSICAL EXAMINATION
The General Inspection

Look for a head tilt, which can be observed in superior oblique palsy (where the patient tilts the head to the unaffected side to minimize diplopia) or in central and peripheral vestibular disorders.[9] Vertical misalignment of the eyes in the absence of an extraocular muscle palsy (skew deviation) can occur in peripheral and central vestibular loss but is thought more common in the latter and has been identified as a useful discriminator in the separation of central and peripheral causes of acute vestibular syndrome.[10] Ocular tilt reaction (OTR) refers to the triad of skew deviation, head tilt (toward the hypotropic eye), and ocular counter-roll (**Fig. 1**). These 3 findings are attributed to a unilateral lesion of the so-called graviceptive pathways arising from the utricle. A vestibular or lower brainstem lesion causes an ipsiversive OTR. To check for skew deviation, a cover test should be performed. When each eye is covered in turn (alternate cover test), a corrective vertical saccade occurs in the uncovered eye, bringing the hypotropic (down) eye upwards or the hypertropic (up) eye downwards. The head tilt in OTR is toward the lower eye (see **Fig. 1**)

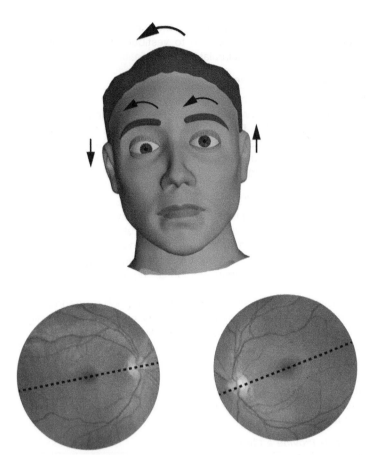

Fig. 1. Right ocular tilt response. A right-sided ocular tilt response characterized by a right head tilt, skew deviation with right hypotropia, and left hypertropia, rightward ocular tilt response.

Horner syndrome (unilateral ptosis, miosis, anhydrosis, and enophthalmos) is caused by lesions affecting sympathetic pathways and must be sought especially in patients with acute vestibular syndrome, because it can accompany brainstem strokes (for example, lateral medullary infarction). The pupillary asymmetry enhances in dim light; therefore, comparison of pupil size in the light and darkness is helpful.

Inspection for Spontaneous and Gaze-evoked Nystagmus

Vestibular vertigo is often associated with spontaneous nystagmus that could point to its origin. First, observe the eyes as the subject fixes on a target and look for primary position spontaneous nystagmus and saccadic intrusions. Next, observe the effect of leftward and rightward gaze (15° from the primary position). Saccadic intrusions are fast eye movements that take the eye away from the primary position. They include square wave jerks, which are minute saccades (0.5°–3°, separated by an approximately 2000-ms interval) that make the eye oscillate to and from the primary position (common in cerebellar disease and extrapyramidal disorders); ocular flutters, which are high-frequency (10–15 Hz) showers of horizontal saccades without an interval; and opsoclonus, which are flurries of vertical, horizontal, and torsional oscillations typically seen in infectious, paraneoplastic, and toxic pathologies affecting the brainstem and cerebellum.

Spontaneous nystagmus arising from an acute peripheral vestibular loss (eg, from vestibular neuritis) gives rise to horizontal torsional nystagmus that beats away from the lesioned ear (**Fig. 2**, Video 1). The nystagmus is unidirectional and maximal when gazing in the direction of the fast phase (Alexander's law) and suppresses with visual fixation (see **Figs. 2** and **3**, Videos 1–3). To ensure spontaneous nystagmus is not missed, visual fixation must be removed. This can be done using a pair of optical or video Frenzel glasses (takeaway Frenzels)[11] or using a penlight test. To do this, the examiner could cover 1 eye and shine a penlight torch directly on the uncovered eye, thus removing visual fixation. Nystagmus intensity is then compared for the illuminated eye with the cover on and off.[12] Failure to remove visual fixation might cause spontaneous nystagmus to be missed. Examining a dizzy patient without some means of removing visual fixation is like trying to auscultate the heart without a stethoscope.

Typical central nystagmus could be bidirectional (left beating on left gaze, rights beating on rightward gaze), vertical (primary position upbeat or downbeat), or purely torsional. Although all these features immediately imply a central cause for acute vertigo, the converse is not true (ie, typical peripheral nystagmus that is horizontal-torsional, is unidirectional, and that suppresses with fixation does not assure the clinician of an underlying peripheral cause because it can often be seen in central vertigo, including cerebellar infarction and vestibular migraine).

Horizontal gaze-evoked nystagmus (see Video 3) is commonly encountered as a by-product of anticonvulsant, lithium, or alcohol intoxication or brainstem (vestibular nucleus or nucleus prepositus hypoglossi) or cerebellar disorders.

Provocative Testing for Positional Nystagmus

Positional testing holds the key to the diagnosis of BPV, which is the most common and correctable cause of vertigo worldwide. For example, in a patient with left

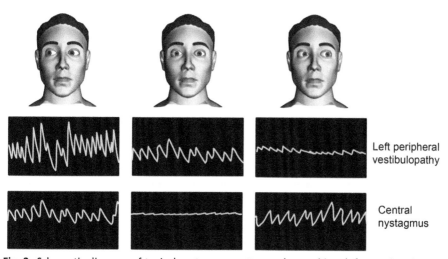

Left peripheral vestibulopathy

Central nystagmus

Fig. 2. Schematic diagram of typical nystagmus patterns observed in a left peripheral vestibulopathy and in cerebellar pathology. The top panel shows typical peripheral right-beating nystagmus that is unidirectional and enhances on rightward gaze. The bottom panel shows typical gaze-evoked nystagmus, which beats leftward on left gaze and rightward on right gaze.

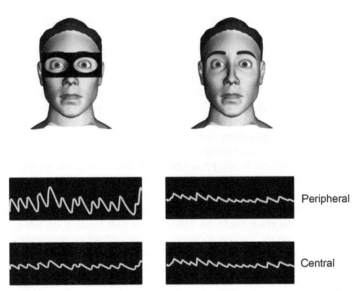

Fig. 3. Visual suppression of nystagmus. Typical peripheral nystagmus amplifies when the subject dons a pair of Frenzel goggles (*top panel*) and is suppressed in bright light. Central nystagmus is unaffected by visual fixation.

posterior canal BPV, in the upright position, the duct of the posterior canal aligns with earth vertical and the otoconia gravitate toward the lowermost part of the duct to lie close to the ampulla (**Fig. 4**A). When the head is rotated 45° to the left and rapidly pitched backwards, the otoconia move along the left posterior canal to lie midway along the duct (see **Fig. 4**B). The resultant plunger effect or negative pressure causes ampullofugal movement of the cupula and briefly excites the posterior canal afferents, producing the characteristic paroxysm of upbeat torsional geotropic nystagmus (where the upper pole of the eye torts toward the lowermost ear) that is the hallmark of posterior canal BPV (Video 4).

Horizontal canal BPV is a far less common cause of positional vertigo and is best evoked by the supine roll test. The subject begins by assuming the supine position, lying on a single pillow, with the head elevated 30° from horizontal, to align the horizontal canals with earth vertical. Consider right horizontal canalithiasis where rotating to the affected right side provokes a paroxysm of horizontal geotropic nystagmus beating toward the right side (**Fig. 5**B, Video 5). Rotation to the left provokes a similar but less intense paroxysm to the left. Lying face down from an initial upright position or pitching the head down provokes horizontal right-beating nystagmus and lying supine provokes left-beating nystagmus. To correctly identify the affected ear, nystagmus intensity with either ear down can be compared. If an examiner has access to video goggles, supine (contraversive) and prone (ipsiversive) nystagmus also helps identify the affected side.[13]

Persistent, direction-changing horizontal positional nystagmus is observed in horizontal canal BPV secondary to cupulolithiasis, where otoconia are adherent to the horizontal canal cupula. In contrast to horizontal canalithiasis, the positional nystagmus is apogeotropic, meaning that the nystagmus beats away from the lowermost ear during supine testing. The nystagmus is more pronounced with the unaffected ear down.[13] Persistent geotropic and apogeotropic horizontal positional nystagmus can also be seen in central vestibular disorders, inclusive of vestibular migraine (Video 6).[13]

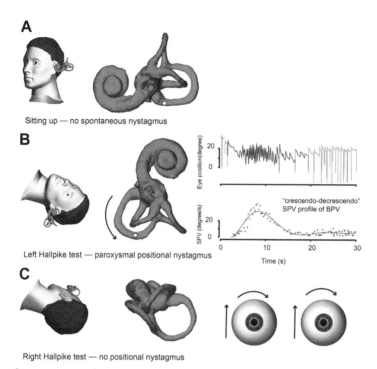

A

Sitting up — no spontaneous nystagmus

B

"crescendo-decrescendo"
SPV profile of BPV

Left Hallpike test — paroxysmal positional nystagmus

Time (s)

C

Right Hallpike test — no positional nystagmus

Fig. 4. Left posterior canal BPV. (*A*) In the upright subject, the otoconia lie in the lowermost part of the left posterior canal. No spontaneous nystagmus is seen. (*B*) As the head is turned 45° to the left and lowered to the Hallpike position, otoconia drift downward (ampullofugally). Ampullofugal movement of the cupula excites vertical canal afferents. Left posterior canal afferents are activated, briefly resulting in a paroxysm of upbeat geotropic torsional nystagmus consistent with left posterior canal BPV. The panels on the right side illustrate eye position and nystagmus slow-phase velocity in the vertical plane, with a crescendo-decrescendo profile. (*From* Lechner C. Open Your Eyes! Video-oculography findings in benign positional vertigo masters of philosophy [thesis]. University of Sydney. 2015; with permission.)

Anterior canal BPV is rare and is also elicited with a Hallpike test. Left anterior canal BPV could result in a positive right or left Hallpike test. The nystagmus, regardless of which ear is down, is downbeat, with a torsional component that beats to the affected left side (Video 7). Anterior canal BPV is so rare that torsional downbeat nystagmus on positional testing should raise the possibility of an underlying central cause, unless the nystagmus abolishes after a successful liberatory maneuver.

Spontaneous nystagmus can enhance in the supine position, leading to an incorrect diagnosis of positional vertigo. For example, a subject with left vestibular neuritis could demonstrate dramatic enhancement of subtle right-beating nystagmus in either Hallpike position. If the primary position spontaneous nystagmus is missed (during examination in a brightly lit emergency department), then enhanced spontaneous nystagmus could be mistaken for BPV and inappropriately treated with repositioning maneuvers, which would only lead to increasing nausea and motion sensitivity. Enhanced spontaneous nystagmus distinctly differs from BPV in that it is persistent rather than paroxysmal and is unidirectional (for example, right-beating nystagmus is observed with the right ear down and the left ear down).

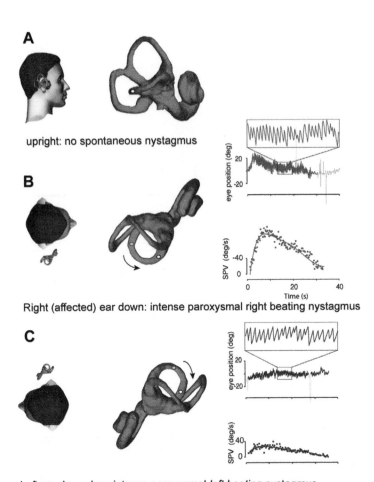

Fig. 5. Right horizontal canal BPV. (*A*) In the upright subject, otoconia lie along the lowest part of the duct of the horizontal canal. No spontaneous nystagmus is seen. When lying on the affected right side, the otoconia drift ampullopetally. For the horizontal canals, ampullopetal movement of the cupula constitutes excitation and excitatory right-beating nystagmus follows. The panel on the right side illustrates eye position and slow-phase velocity as a function of time. The nystagmus slow-phase velocity shows the typical rise and fall. When lying on the unaffected left side, the otoconia drift ampullofugally and inhibit the right horizontal anal afferents, and inhibitory (left-beating) nystagmus follows. The nystagmus profiles with the affected and unaffected ears down are similar but the peak velocity is higher with the affected ear down. The side with the more pronounced nystagmus is considered the affected side. (*From* Lechner C. Open Your Eyes! Video-oculography findings in benign positional vertigo masters of philosophy [thesis]. University of Sydney. 2015; with permission.)

Head-shaking nystagmus

Head-shaking nystagmus is an additional method of demonstrating a left-right asymmetry in dynamic vestibular function. While wearing Frenzel glasses, the patient's head is bent slightly forwards (30°) to align the horizontal canals with earth horizontal. The head is shaken in the yaw plane at 2 per second approximately 10 to 20 times. If there is a unilateral vestibular lesion, horizontal nystagmus with the quick phases beating to the intact ear (contraversive head-shaking nystagmus) is seen at the end of head shaking. Nystagmus may reverse thereafter. Normal subjects have no head-shaking nystagmus or only 1 to 2 beats. Vertical nystagmus observed after horizontal head shaking is a nonspecific sign, thought to imply central vestibulopathy. Ipsiversive head-shaking nystagmus (with the fast phase beating toward the lesioned ear) has been described in lateral medullary infarction.[14]

The Head Impulse

The head impulse test is a simple and effective method of assessing the integrity of the horizontal vestibulo-ocular reflex (VOR) and is indispensable in the assessment of the acute vestibular syndrome.[15] It is within the capability of any clinician, but like any part of the neurologic examination it is a skill acquired after much practice. To perform the head impulse test, the patient fixates on a target approximately 1 m away. The examiner firmly grasps the patient's head with both hands and turns it briskly to the left or the right (**Fig. 6**). The impulses should be unpredictable, low-amplitude (10°–20°), high-acceleration (2000°–4000° /s²) movements. When the VOR is intact, each head movement is associated with an equal and opposite eye movement, thus maintaining visual fixation on the target (see **Figs. 6**B, C). When the VOR is impaired unilaterally, a head impulse to the affected side causes the head and eyes to initially move together,

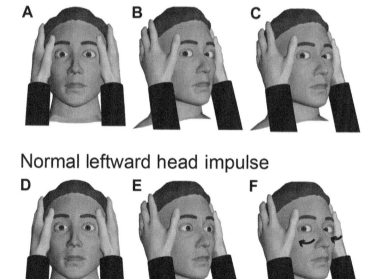

Normal leftward head impulse

Positive leftward head impulse

Fig. 6. The head impulse test. The top panel illustrates a normal (negative) head impulse test. The subject fixes on a near target (the examiner's nose). (*A*) When the head is turned left, the intact left horizontal VOR produces an equal and opposite eye movement that returns the eye to the target (*B*, *C*). The bottom panel shows a VOR deficit. (*E*) When the head is turned leftward, the eyes initially move with the head. (*F*) A refixation saccade, or catch-up saccade, returns the eye back to the target.

followed by a rapid corrective eye movement or catch-up saccade, which rapidly refixates the eye (see **Fig. 6**F). A positive catch-up saccade in the horizontal canal plane is usually evident in the subject presenting with an acute vestibular syndrome secondary to superior vestibular neuritis.[3,10,15]

To confidently separate vestibular neuritis from an acute vestibular syndrome of central origin, it is essential to demonstrate a positive HINTS plus battery test (horizontal head, impulse test, typical peripheral nystagmus, absence of skew deviation, and normal hearing), shown to separate central from peripheral causes of acute vestibular syndrome.[16] Sometimes, despite a significant horizontal canal deficit, the catch-up saccade is not detectable at the bedside, because it actually occurs while the head is still moving. These saccades, evident only on video head-impulse testing, are covert saccades.[17]

Oculomotor Examination

Test horizontal and vertical saccades

Saccades are rapid eye movements that point the fovea at an object of interest. To test saccades, ask the patient to rapidly fixate on 2 stationary objects (clinician's thumb and index finger) placed 50 cm apart and observe saccadic latency, velocity, accuracy, and conjugacy. Saccadic abnormalities are not expected in peripheral vestibular disorders. Slow saccades of restricted amplitude may reflect an ocular muscle or ocular motor nerve paresis. Disconjugate slowing of horizontal saccades is an abnormality observed in internuclear ophthalmoplegia, which is caused by lesions affecting the median longitudinal fasciculus (MLF). A unilateral MLF lesion results in selective slowing of adducting saccades on testing horizontal saccades to the unaffected side. The abducting eye may sometimes demonstrate disconjugate nystagmus (ie, the nystagmus is more marked in the abducting than the adducting eye). In an acutely dizzy patient, an internuclear ophthalmoplegia might imply a brainstem stroke or demyelination. Saccadic dysmetria, in particular hypermetria, is seen in cerebellar disease. The saccade overshoots and returns to the target. Ipsipulsion, with hypermetria of ipsilateral saccades and hypometria of contralateral saccades, occurs in a lateral medullary infarct and is due to interruption of olivocerebellar climbing fibers in the inferior cerebellar peduncle and downstream inhibition of the ipsilateral fastigial nucleus.

Test pursuit

To test smooth pursuit, ask the patient to follow an object (clinician's finger) moving no faster than 20° per second in both the horizontal and vertical directions. Look for broken or saccadic pursuit. Because many parts of the neuraxis participate in smooth pursuit, broken pursuit does not contribute greatly to identifying the site of a lesion. Age, level of alertness, intoxication, and neurodegenerative disorders affecting the cerebellum and basal ganglia can all impair smooth pursuit. Deficits in smooth pursuit are usually accompanied by impaired visual cancellation of the VOR.

Visual cancellation of the vestibulo-ocular reflex

Ask the patient to sit on a swivel chair with arms extended, hands clasped and thumbs pointing up. Rotate the patient en bloc in the yaw plane as the patient fixes on his/her own thumbs. Inspect the eyes for quick phases. In a normal subject with normal VOR cancellation, the eyes remain fixed on the target and no quick phases are observed. In cerebellar disorders and in disorders of smooth pursuit, VOR cancellation is impaired and quick phases toward the direction of rotation are observed.

Vestibulospinal Reflexes

Vision, proprioception, and vestibulospinal contributions enable upright stance; therefore, disturbances in any one of these contributors can affect gait and stance. Patients with an acute unilateral vestibulopathy typically fall toward the side of the lesion. In the acute vestibular syndrome, inability to maintain upright stance with the eyes open should raise the possibility of a cerebellar infarct. Examine the patient's normal gait, then the tandem gait forward and backward. Look for a wide-based gait, which can be observed in a cerebellar disorder but is not specific for it. Perform the standard Romberg test, where the patient stands on flat ground with a normal stance width, with the eyes shut; vestibular impairment does not cause a positive Romberg test when proprioception is intact. Ask the patient to stand on a 20-cm thick foam cushion, which interrupts proprioceptive information and causes inability to maintain upright stance in subjects with bilateral vestibular loss. The Unterberger test is performed by asking the patient to march in place with eyes closed for 30 seconds and noting any excessive turning to the side of vestibular impairment.

General Neurologic Assessment

As with any other patient presenting with neurologic symptoms, a general neurologic examination inclusive of a search for lateralizing cranial nerve signs, long tract signs, cerebellar ataxia, and sensory loss should be undertaken.

Postural Blood Pressure, Pulse, and Auscultation

Lying and standing blood pressure and pulse measurement (20-mm systolic blood pressure drop or 30 beats per minute heart rate rise) help identify orthostatic intolerance as a cause of dizziness. Auscultation of the heart, neck, and supraclavicular fossa is important to detect vascular bruits and cardiac murmurs that might be linked with either lightheadedness (eg, aortic stenosis) or vertigo (eg, subclavian steal).

WHAT MIGHT BE SEEN IN A PATIENT PRESENTING WITH ACUTE VESTIBULAR SYNDROME
Vestibular Neuritis

Vestibular neuritis is associated with horizontal torsional nystagmus that is unidirectional, beats away from the affected ear, suppresses with visual fixation, and is maximal on gazing in the direction of the quick phase. The nystagmus enhances dramatically with either Hallpike test (if the patient allows the clinician to do this). A positive horizontal head impulse test is seen on turning toward the lesioned side, with a rapid corrective saccade or catch-up saccade. Hearing is uniformly normal in vestibular neuritis. Abnormal hearing in the context of an acute vestibular syndrome could imply an AICA infarction. An ipsilateral ocular tilt response rarely occurs in vestibular neuritis, with head tilt toward the affected ear, skew deviation with hypotropia on the side of the ear, and ocular torsion toward the side of the lesion. Because skew deviation in the context of vertigo is seen more commonly with posterior circulation strokes, it is considered a red flag for central vertigo.

Cerebellar Stroke

Although typical cerebellar nystagmus is bidirectional (left beating on left gaze and right beating on right gaze), cerebellar strokes can present with second- or third-degree spontaneous horizontal nystagmus (typical peripheral nystagmus).[18] Typical cerebellar nystagmus (see Video 2) is attributed to abnormalities in the cerebellar flocculus (vestibulocerebellum) or the medial vestibular nucleus-nucleus prepositus hypoglossus complex in the medulla. The head impulse test is negative except in AICA infarcts and skew deviation may be evident. In recent studies by Chen and colleagues,[19] 62% of subjects with AICA infarcts had positive clinical head impulse tests ipsilateral to the infarct. Even 20% of posterior inferior cerebellar artery/superior cerebellar artery infarcts had a contralaterally positive clinical head impulses. On quantitative testing, the amplitude of catch-up saccades observed in vestibular neuritis were twice as large. In cases of an AICA infarct, hearing loss is evident on the side with concurrent vestibular loss. Saccadic dysmetria, unilateral deficits in VOR suppression, or appendicular cerebellar signs might help, but the key to identifying stroke is the failure to pass the HINTS battery. In patients with an acute vestibular syndrome, any one of the following attributes should trigger a search for cerebellar stroke: a normal head impulse, presence of skew, cerebellar nystagmus, or a new hearing loss.

WHAT MIGHT BE SEEN IN EPISODIC SPONTANEOUS VERTIGO
Meniere Disease

An episode of acute vertigo in Meniere disease is characterized by typical peripheral nystagmus that is unidirectional, obeys Alexander's law, and is enhanced in the dark. In contrast to other peripheral vestibular disorders, the nystagmus could first beat toward the affected ear (irritative nystagmus), within seconds to minutes change direction to beat toward the unaffected ear (paretic nystagmus) (Video 8),[20,21] and finally change direction once more (recovery nystagmus) to beat to the affected ear. This sequence of direction change in primary position spontaneous nystagmus has only been reported in endolymphatic hydrops.

Vestibular Migraine

An acutely dizzy patient with vestibular migraine could present with spontaneous horizontal, vertical, or pure torsional nystagmus.[22] Additionally both horizontal and vertical positional nystagmus can be observed in vestibular migraine. In contrast to BPV, the positional nystagmus of vestibular migraine is persistent and remains as long as the head remains in the provocative position (see Video 6).[23] When the nystagmus is horizontal, both geotropic and apogeotropic positional nystagmus can be observed.[13,23]

WHAT MIGHT BE SEEN IN THE PATIENT WITH RECURRENT POSITIONAL VERTIGO
Benign Positional Vertigo

Typical posterior canal BPV is not associated with primary position spontaneous nystagmus; during Hallpike testing with the affected ear down, paroxysmal positional nystagmus with a vertical upbeating torsional geotropic eye movement is observed (see **Fig. 4**, Video 4). The nystagmus could begin after a 5- to 10-second latency and rapidly rises to a crescendo, completely abating by 60 seconds. Hallpike testing with the unaffected ear down generally yields no nystagmus but rarely could produce low-amplitude nystagmus similar to that observed with the affected ear down. Returning the patient from the Hallpike position to an upright position causes reverse flow of otoconia (ampullopetally) and torsional downbeat nystagmus with torsion toward the unaffected ear. Horizontal canal BPV, anterior canal BPV, and central vestibular disorders can also present with recurrent positional vertigo. Annotated videos of these less common presentations of positional vertigo are included (see Videos 5–7).

WHEN THE PATIENT IS ACUTELY DIZZY AND THERE ARE NO PHYSICAL SIGNS TO FIND

Failure to demonstrate nystagmus in a brightly lit room is of no diagnostic value. In an acutely dizzy patient, however, the absence of nystagmus when examined without visual fixation implies a nonvestibular cause for vertigo. Consider hypotension, cardiac rhythm disturbances, hypoglycemia, anemia, and anxiety, especially if associated with other panic symptoms and reproducible with hyperventilation.

FUTURE DIRECTIONS IN ACUTE VERTIGO

A majority of acutely vertiginous patients present to an emergency department and general practice rather than a specialty clinic. Frontline practitioners have the unique opportunity of observing ictal nystagmus, which provides critical information that could streamline the diagnostic process, but they lack the expertise and the equipment to elicit, record, or interpret nystagmus. Conversely, expert clinicians who have all of these seldom have the opportunity of assessing an acutely vertiginous patient. The use of inexpensive methods of removing visual fixation[11] and portable video recording devices in emergency departments and general practice settings could correct this discrepancy. In an era when many adults own a handheld device with a digital camera, it is inconceivable that a general practitioner or emergency physician has no access to a simple video Frenzel device or its equivalent. Easy access to the correct tools and greater familiarity with cardinal eye signs of common vestibular disorders promote early diagnosis and better management of acutely dizzy patients in the frontline.

SUPPLEMENTARY DATA

Supplementary data related to this article can be found online at http://dx.doi.org/10.1016/j.ncl.2015.04.001.

REFERENCES

1. Newman-Toker DE, Cannon LM, Stofferahn ME, et al. Imprecision in patient reports of dizziness symptom quality: a cross-sectional study conducted in an acute care setting. Mayo Clin Proc 2007;82:1329–40.
2. Jeong SH, Kim HJ, Kim JS. Vestibular neuritis. Semin Neurol 2013;33(3):185–94.
3. Kattah JC, Talkad AV, Wang DZ, et al. HINTS to diagnose stroke in the acute vestibular syndrome: three-step bedside oculo motor examination more sensitive than early MRdiffusion-weighted imaging. Stroke 2009;40:3504–10.
4. Furman JM, Marcus DA, Balaban CD. Vestibular migraine: clinical aspects and pathophysiology. Lancet Neurol 2013;12(7):706–15.
5. Hüfner K, Barresi D, Glaser M, et al. Vestibular paroxysmia: diagnostic features and medical treatment. Neurology 2008;71(13):1006–14.
6. Lee H, Ahn BH, Baloh RW. Sudden deafness with vertigo as a sole manifestation of anterior inferior cerebellar artery infarction. J Neurol Sci 2004;222(1–2):105–7.
7. Hamid MA. Ménière's disease. Pract Neurol 2009;9(3):157–62.
8. Fife TD, Giza C. Posttraumatic vertigo and dizziness. Semin Neurol 2013;33(3):238–43.
9. Brandt T, Dieterich M. Skew deviation with ocular torsion: a vestibular brainstem sign of topographic diagnostic value. Ann Neurol 1993;33(5):528–34.
10. Cnyrim CD, Newman-Toker D, Karch C, et al. Bedside differentiation of vestibular neuritis from central "vestibular pseudoneuritis". J Neurol Neurosurg Psychiatry 2008;79(4):458–60.

11. Strupp M, Fischer C, Hanß L, et al. The takeaway Frenzel goggles: a Fresnel-based device. Neurology 2014;83(14):1241–5.
12. Newman-Toker DE, Sharma P, Chowdhury M, et al. Penlight-cover test: a new bedside method to unmask nystagmus. J Neurol Neurosurg Psychiatry 2009; 80:900–3.
13. Lechner C, Taylor RL, Todd C, et al. Causes and characteristics of horizontal positional nystagmus. J Neurol 2014;261(5):1009–17.
14. Choi KD, Oh SY, Park SH, et al. Head-shaking nystagmus in lateral medullary infarction: patterns and possible mechanisms. Neurology 2007;68(17):1337–44.
15. Halmagyi GM, Curthoys IS. A clinical sign of canal paresis. Arch Neurol 1988; 45(7):737–94.
16. Tarnutzer AA, Berkowitz AL, Robinson KA, et al. Does my dizzy patient have a stroke? A systematic review of bedside diagnosis in acute vestibular syndrome. CMAJ 2011;183(9):E571–92.
17. Weber KP, Aw ST, Todd MJ, et al. Head impulse test in unilateral vestibular loss: vestibulo-ocular reflex and catch-up saccades. Neurology 2008;70(6):454–63.
18. Lee H, Sohn SI, Cho YW, et al. Cerebellar infarction presenting isolated vertigo: frequency and vascular topographical patterns. Neurology 2006;67(7):1178–83.
19. Chen L, Todd M, Halmagyi GM, et al. Head impulse gain and saccade analysis in pontine-cerebellar stroke and vestibular neuritis. Neurology 2014;83(17): 1513–22.
20. Bance M, Mai M, Tomlinson D, et al. The changing direction of nystagmus in acute Ménière's disease: pathophysiological implications. Laryngoscope 1991; 101(2):197–201.
21. McClure JA, Copp JC, Lycett P. Recovery nystagmus in Ménière's disease. Laryngoscope 1981;91(10):1727–37.
22. von Brevern M, Zeise D, Neuhauser H, et al. Acute migrainous vertigo: clinical and oculographic findings. Brain 2005;128(Pt 2):365–74.
23. Lechner C. Open Your Eyes! Video-oculography findings in benign positional vertigo masters of philosophy [thesis]. University of Sydney; 2015.

Misdiagnosing Dizzy Patients
Common Pitfalls in Clinical Practice

 CrossMark

Kevin A. Kerber, MD, MS[a,*], David E. Newman-Toker, MD, PhD[b]

KEYWORDS

- Dizziness • Vestibular disorder • Vertigo • Management

KEY POINTS

- Opportunities exist to improve the diagnosis and management of patients with acute dizziness in routine care settings.
- To optimize the accuracy and efficiency of diagnosis in acute dizziness and vertigo, providers should deemphasize the type of dizziness, patient demographics, and the routine use of computed tomography (or MRI) neuroimaging.
- Providers should emphasize the timing and triggers for dizziness symptoms and leverage bedside eye movement assessments to identify opportunities to effectively and efficiently diagnose and treat common peripheral vestibular disorders and simultaneously to determine whether MRI neuroimaging is indicated to search for dangerous central causes.

INTRODUCTION

As a general rule, peripheral vestibular disorders are not correctly diagnosed or managed in the emergency department (ED), with misdiagnosis rates estimated in the range of 74% to 81%.[1,2] Common disorders such as benign paroxysmal positional vertigo (BPPV) and vestibular neuritis are frequently confused for one another[1] and for more serious central causes such as stroke.[2] Management is non–evidence based and suboptimal.[3,4]

Identifying peripheral vestibular disorders should be a priority for several reasons. First, these disorders are very common; BPPV alone has an estimated lifetime prevalence around 2%.[5] Second, evidence-based treatments exist. The most common peripheral vestibular disorder, BPPV, has systematic reviews and clinical guideline

[a] Department of Neurology, University of Michigan Health System, 1500 East Medical Center Drive, Ann Arbor, MI 48109, USA; [b] Departments of Neurology and Otolaryngology Head and Neck Surgery, Johns Hopkins Hospital, The Johns Hopkins University School of Medicine & Bloomberg School of Public Health, CRB-II, Room 2M-03 North, 1550 Orleans Street, Baltimore, MD 21231, USA
* Corresponding author.
E-mail address: kakerber@umich.edu

Neurol Clin 33 (2015) 565–575
http://dx.doi.org/10.1016/j.ncl.2015.04.009
0733-8619/15/$ – see front matter © 2015 Elsevier Inc. All rights reserved.
neurologic.theclinics.com

statements to support the use of the Dix-Hallpike test and the highly effective canalith repositioning maneuver.[6,7] Physical therapy strategies are also supported by systematic reviews for the treatment of acute unilateral vestibulopathy (eg, vestibular neuritis).[8] Optimal identification of peripheral vestibular disorders could enable more efficient care because additional laboratory or imaging tests are not necessary and are generally not even warranted in the management of these disorders.[6] In addition, physicians who can accurately identify peripheral vestibular disorders are probably better equipped to identify dangerous central vestibular disorders because the probability of a central disorder substantially increases when peripheral vestibular disorders are ruled out.

Identifying central vestibular disorders is also important. Vascular causes (stroke or transient ischemic attack [TIA]) are the most common central disorders that present with acute dizziness[9] and evidence-based treatments exist for both acute and chronic management to improve functional recovery and reduce the risk for future stroke events.[10] Clinical practice research suggests that identifying stroke-dizziness presentations may be suboptimal. One population-based study found that 16 out of 46 (35%) acute stroke/TIA-dizziness cases did not receive a stroke or TIA diagnosis from the treating ED provider.[11] Dizziness was also found to be the presenting symptom most closely linked with subsequent stroke presentations in the ED, a finding that suggests the initial dizziness presentations may have been misdiagnosed as nonvascular events.[12] In another population-based study, TIAs presenting posterior circulation symptoms such as isolated dizziness and vertigo were initially misdiagnosed in 90% of cases (n = 9 out of 10).[13]

Harm may result from missed opportunities to apply timely therapies for underlying disorders, including both peripheral and central diseases. For example, patients with BPPV who are not treated within 24 hours of the ED visit have more than double the recurrence risk (46% vs 20%; P = .002)[14] and unrecognized BPPV confers 6.5-fold greater odds of falling.[15] When stroke diagnosis is delayed, missed opportunities for thrombolysis,[16] early surgery for complications such as malignant posterior fossa edema,[17] and early prevention of subsequent vertebrobasilar infarction can result in permanent disability or death.

This article explores some of the likely reasons why misdiagnosis is frequent. It highlights 5 diagnostic pitfalls (Table 1) often encountered in clinical practice, and makes recommendations for how to avoid these known traps when assessing acutely dizzy patients.

PITFALL 1: OVERRELIANCE ON THE TYPE OF DIZZINESS TO GUIDE DIAGNOSTIC INQUIRY

The traditional approach to the evaluation of patients who present with dizziness symptoms has been to heavily weight defining the type of symptom when assessing the most likely cause.[18,19] The recommended first question for the patient is generally, "What do you mean by dizzy?" In this traditional paradigm, the dizziness is classified into one of 4 specific types: (1) vertigo (the illusion of spinning or other false motion); (2) presyncope (a feeling of impending faint or loss of consciousness); (3) disequilibrium or loss of balance without head sensation; and (4) other ill-defined symptoms such as lightheadedness, wooziness, or giddiness.[18] The teaching suggests that once a patient is categorized as having a type of dizziness, the likely causes are as follows: vertigo, which is thought to indicate a vestibular disorder; presyncope, which indicates a cardiovascular disorder; disequilibrium, which indicates a neurologic disorder; and nonspecific dizziness, which indicates a psychiatric or metabolic disorder.[19]

Table 1
Summary of common pitfalls in current approaches to diagnosing acute dizziness

Pitfalls	Additional Information
1. Overreliance on type of dizziness to guide diagnostic inquiry	Patients' descriptions of symptom type are not reliable Types of dizziness are not valid discriminators The type of dizziness should be deemphasized when making diagnostic and management decisions
2. Underuse and misuse of timing and triggers to categorize patients for diagnosis	Patients' report of timing and triggers are reliable Major causes of dizziness have characteristic timing and triggers, so these attributes should be emphasized Care should be taken to distinguish triggers from exacerbating features, which have different implications for diagnosis
3. Underuse, misuse, and misconceptions linked to hallmark eye examination findings	Major causes of dizziness have hallmark eye movement examination findings that are virtually pathognomonic Frontline providers and neurologists should be better trained in the use of these hallmark examination findings
4. Overweighting age, vascular risk factors, and neuroexamination to screen for stroke	Although older patients with vascular risk factors are more likely to have stroke as a cause for dizziness or vertigo, young patients with stroke are far more likely to be missed, with potentially serious consequences Patients with central patterns of eye movements are still at a very high risk of acute stroke even when there are no vascular risk factors or general neurologic abnormalities
5. Overuse and overreliance on head CT to rule out neurologic causes	Head CT is commonly and increasingly used in acute presentations of dizziness. Head CT is an insensitive test for acute ischemic stroke, which is the most common central cause of acute dizziness, so its use should be severely curtailed If neuroimaging is required, MRI-DWI is the test of choice

Abbreviations: CT, computed tomography; DWI, diffusion-weighted imaging.

This symptom type approach has frequently been endorsed in the medical literature.[20] Studies confirm that frontline physicians consider the type of dizziness to be very important. A survey of more than 400 ED physicians revealed consensus that the approach to dizziness based on the type of symptom is the dominant method presented in the medical literature and teaching, and roughly 90% personally endorse this approach.[20] When asked to rank the relative importance of several symptom attributes to diagnostic assessment of a patient with dizziness in the ED, most physicians (64%) ranked symptom type first; roughly 5-fold more often than the next nearest attribute. Most (69%) respondents agreed that they do not pursue cardiovascular causes if the patient reports vertigo, or vestibular causes if the patient reports presyncope, indicating that they make clinical decisions based on the type of symptom, including when not to pursue diagnoses.[20]

The problem with the type of dizziness being used as the principal factor in the diagnostic process is that it is neither a reliable symptom attribute reported by patients nor a valid discriminator among different causes of dizziness.[21,22] Low reliability of patient reports of the type of dizziness was shown by research that queried patients presenting to the ED regarding dizziness symptoms that included a test-retest paradigm.[21] Of more than 300 patients with dizziness interviewed, more than half changed their choice of the best descriptor for their dizziness when asked the same question 5 to 10 minutes after their initial selection. Furthermore, patients' open-ended descriptions of dizziness were often vague, circular, or hard to understand, making them difficult to categorize using the traditional paradigm. Examples of responses to the question "What do you mean by 'dizzy'?" included the following: "Yes, like your head is becoming empty," and "I think the general meaning would be the point where that woozy feeling; now I don't know how you want to describe the adjective for that; I guess woozy at that point."

Categorizing patients based on the type of dizziness is also problematic because patients typically use more than one type of dizziness to describe their symptoms. Patients allowed to choose from a list of 6 types of dizziness to describe their symptoms selected an average of 2.6 types, with nearly 80% selecting more than 1 type and 50% selecting 3 or more types.[21] Roughly 75% of those who selected a descriptor other than vertigo answered directed questions about false spinning or motion that indicated that they were experiencing vertigo. It is therefore difficult to imagine how the type of dizziness could possibly inform the differential diagnosis for the underlying cause.

Regarding the validity of the type of dizziness as a discriminator among causes, systematic reviews have found no published studies that support the predictive validity of the symptom type.[22,23] Small studies have shown no association between dizziness type and eventual clinical diagnoses (eg, type of dizziness fails to adequately differentiate central from peripheral causes[24] or psychiatric from vestibular causes[25]).

Reliability and validity of information gathered are the cornerstones of diagnostic evaluation. Factors shown to not be adequately reliable or valid should be downgraded rather than emphasized when formulating a diagnosis and planning the evaluation and management. In this case, the type or quality of dizziness symptoms should be given little or no diagnostic weight.

PITFALL 2: UNDERUSE AND MISUSE OF TIMING AND TRIGGERS TO CATEGORIZE PATIENTS FOR DIAGNOSIS

Frontline providers typically overemphasize symptom types, and they also usually underemphasize or misuse timing and triggers in dizziness,[26] which are aspects that are more reliably reported by patients and thus can be used to more effectively categorize clinical presentations.[21] In contrast with the low reliability of patient descriptions of the type of dizziness, patients have been shown to be reliable in describing the duration and triggers of the dizziness symptoms.[21] Regarding the timing of symptoms (episode duration), 81% of patients report consistent responses on being asked the same question within minutes of the initial question. Similarly, a high proportion of patients (91%–100%) provide consistent responses regarding questions about symptom triggers (ie, postural/positional, head motion, rolling in bed).

The reliability of these features is important because common causes of dizziness, such as BPPV and vestibular neuritis, have hallmark features in terms of their timing and triggers.[27,28] The timing of vestibular symptoms (including episode, relapse, and illness duration; symptom onset; and frequency) has been studied extensively in individual disease populations.[25,29–31] The much higher reliability of timing and triggers compared with dizziness type, coupled with important differences in timing and trigger patterns among common causes of dizziness, should increase the diagnostic utility of this information.

However, there is an important pitfall related to misuse of dizziness trigger information: the tendency of physicians to overemphasize positional aspects of the dizziness symptoms and to presume a benign disorder, typically BPPV, when symptom intensity is associated with positional changes.[32] The problem hinges on the critical (but often unrecognized) distinction between symptoms that are positionally triggered and those that are positionally exacerbated.[28] Positionally triggered dizziness or vertigo is most often caused by BPPV, whereas positionally exacerbated dizziness could be of any cause, because virtually every cause of persistent dizziness (benign or dangerous, peripheral or central) is exacerbated by positional changes and at least partially relieved by remaining completely still. Despite this, 80% of physicians mistakenly endorsed the idea that, in patients with persistent dizziness, head motion causing an exacerbation of symptoms is an indicator of a benign condition.[20] These providers likely give this endorsement because they assume a diagnosis of BPPV whenever the patient reports that head motion contributes to the symptoms, without distinguishing triggers (in true episodic dizziness, from an asymptomatic baseline) from exacerbating features (in continuous, ongoing dizziness). BPPV is specifically characterized by discrete, brief, and high-intensity attacks of dizziness triggered by certain head movements (eg, lying down, rolling over in bed, or looking up).[6] A patient with vestibular neuritis or stroke may report minimal or sometimes no symptoms when lying still, particularly if it is a mild case or if hours or days have passed since the onset, but the return of continuous symptoms during normal head movements usually makes the distinction clear. The overlap of a positional component among various causes of dizziness is why it is critical to correctly identify the characteristic BPPV nystagmus with the Dix-Hallpike test (discussed later).[6]

PITFALL 3: UNDERUSE, MISUSE, AND MISCONCEPTIONS LINKED TO HALLMARK EYE EXAMINATION FINDINGS

In the acute setting, the eye movement examination is often the essential element in discriminating among causes of dizziness because the patterns of eye movements are hallmark features of the various disorders (**Table 2**).[27,33] Emphasizing the examination is important because the history of present illness can overlap among the various causes of dizziness, particularly on the first day of symptoms. Although timing and triggers are reliably reported by patients,[21] a patient with severe BPPV symptoms may be difficult to distinguish from a patient with a mild case of vestibular neuritis or stroke simply based on the timing and triggers, or even using additional details about the clinical scenario. It is common, particularly in the acute setting, for patients with BPPV to report continuous (ie, interictal) low-level dizziness symptoms such as mild unsteadiness or mild nausea[34,35] and they may be restricting head movement such that few paroxysmal attacks have occurred. Patients with vestibular neuritis may first notice their symptoms on awakening and sitting up from bed; a description that closely mimics a typical positional trigger history seen in BPPV. Further, patients with mild vestibular neuritis may report feeling near normal at rest and substantial worsening of symptoms with movement. Frontline clinicians seeing patients in the first 24 to 48 hours do not have the advantage of knowing how the symptoms later evolve. The progression over days to weeks often makes distinguishing these disorders more straightforward: BPPV as numerous brief paroxysmal attacks triggered by typical head movements versus vestibular neuritis as a single prolonged bout with dizziness symptoms aggravated/alleviated in relation to activity.

However, common disorders causing dizziness all have hallmark findings on eye movement examination (see **Table 2**). For example, BPPV can be confidently diagnosed in a matter of minutes when there is no spontaneous or gaze-evoked nystagmus and the Dix-Hallpike test triggers transient upbeat-torsional nystagmus, even if the patient reports a continuous dizziness sensation that might suggest otherwise. This BPPV pattern of nystagmus has been well defined based on the anatomy

Table 2
Common eye movement patterns, their nystagmus characteristics, and typical causes

Pattern Types	Nystagmus Characteristics	Typical Causes
Peripheral vestibular patterns	Upbeat-torsional nystagmus triggered by the Dix-Hallpike test and that is transient (lasting <30 s)	BPPV (posterior canal)[a]
	Dominantly horizontal spontaneous nystagmus (ie, present in primary gaze during routine gaze testing) that is unidirectional (ie, never changes direction with gaze shifts or head shaking) but increases in velocity with gaze in the direction of the nystagmus fast phase and decreases with gaze in the opposite direction	Vestibular neuritis (less commonly caused by a central lesion typically associated with other findings[b])
Central vestibular patterns	Dominantly vertical (upbeat or downbeat) or torsional spontaneous nystagmus (ie, present in primary gaze during routine gaze testing)	Stroke, multiple sclerosis, Chiari malformation, other structural central disorders, medication side effects (eg, antiepileptic medications)
	Dominantly horizontal gaze-evoked direction-changing nystagmus (ie, persistent left beat on left gaze and persistent right beat on right gaze)	
	Nonfatiguing positional downbeat nystagmus triggered by a positional test such as the Dix-Hallpike test	
Physiologic patterns	Few beats of end-gaze nystagmus (nonsustained left-beat nystagmus on far left gaze with symmetric right-beat nystagmus on far right gaze)	Normal variant

[a] The second most common variant of BPPV is the horizontal canal variant, which is characterized by transient horizontal nystagmus (rather than upbeat-torsional nystagmus) triggered by a head turn to either side while lying supine (eg, head turn to right triggers right-beat horizontal nystagmus, head turn to left triggers left-beat horizontal nystagmus).
[b] See Chapters 2, 10, and 11 for information regarding findings suggesting a central vestibular lesion in the presence of unidirectional spontaneous nystagmus.

and physiology relevant to BPPV.[33] Similarly, a central cause of dizziness can be presumed whenever a central pattern of nystagmus (eg, dominantly vertical or torsional spontaneous nystagmus, or gaze-evoked bidirectional nystagmus) is identified. Spontaneous unidirectional nystagmus is typically caused by vestibular neuritis, although additional examination elements are needed in this situation to more confidently distinguish this peripheral vestibular disorder from a central vestibular disorder such as stroke (See Chapters 2, 10, & 11).[36]

Although these features enable a rapid diagnostic assessment, frontline physicians frequently underuse or misinterpret the bedside eye movement examination.[1,4] BPPV and vestibular neuritis should be diagnosed, particularly in the acute setting, by confirming the presence of a characteristic pattern of nystagmus.[6,37] A population-based study of ED dizziness presentations found that a nystagmus assessment was documented in most of the visits (81.3%; 887 of 1091 visits).[1] However, when nystagmus was documented as present, only infrequently were there additional details such as the direction of the nystagmus, its presence in primary gaze versus lateral gaze, or the findings with positional testing. Because of the sparse nystagmus details documented in the medical record, neuro-otology raters were only able to draw inferences about the suspected localization or cause in 5.4% of cases documented as having nystagmus present. The use of the Dix-Hallpike test was rarely documented even when the treating physician recorded a diagnosis of BPPV.[4,5] For patients receiving a peripheral vestibular diagnosis (ie, BPPV or vestibular neuritis) from the treating physician, most of the nystagmus descriptions (81%) were incompatible with the diagnosis rendered by the physician.[1] The most common reason that reported nystagmus findings were against the diagnosis was documentation of nystagmus being absent, because BPPV and neuritis both require a specific nystagmus type to be present. However, even when nystagmus was documented to be present, most of the descriptions were also against the diagnosis rendered.

PITFALL 4: OVERWEIGHTING AGE, VASCULAR RISK FACTORS, AND GENERAL NEUROLOGIC EXAMINATION TO SCREEN FOR STROKE

Because hallmark eye examination findings are underused in clinical evaluation, frontline doctors probably overweight vascular risk factors and the general neurologic examination when considering the possibility of acute stroke. Older age, vascular risk factors, and abnormal neurologic examination findings have been shown to be indicators of patients at higher risk of stroke.[11] Demographic factors increase the pretest probability of stroke in acute dizziness presentations, whereas abnormalities on the general neurologic examination (eg, dysarthria, dysmetria) suggest that the dizziness stems from a central lesion. Nevertheless, a patient with central eye movement abnormalities has a substantial probability of stroke even if there are no vascular risk factors or general neurologic abnormalities.[36] Based on data from a series of 190 cases of acute continuous dizziness, providers relying on the ABCD[2] (age, blood pressure, clinical features of unilateral weakness or speech change, duration of symptoms, diabetes) vascular risk score (an aggregate score based on traditional vascular risk factors and components of the general neurologic examination) to identify stroke would miss nearly 40% of the stroke cases and also overcall stroke in nearly 40% of peripheral vestibular cases.[36] Relying on vascular risk factor stratification is particularly likely to miss younger patients with stroke and research suggests that younger patients with dizziness may be more at risk for stroke misdiagnosis than are older patients.[12,36]

The presence of other neurologic symptoms or signs is a strong predictor for a central nervous system cause; typically stroke.[22,38] However, the converse is not necessarily true. Isolated dizziness and vertigo presentations are the most common initial manifestation of posterior circulation (vertebrobasilar) ischemia,[13] and roughly 80% of strokes with the principal symptom of acute continuous dizziness do not have abnormalities on the general neurologic examination.[39] When patients with stroke have a National Institutes of Health stroke scale score of zero, it is often a posterior circulation stroke presenting dizziness, vertigo, or nausea as the chief symptom.[40] Thus, the absence of typical neurologic symptoms or signs suggesting central nervous system involvement should not be relied on to exclude stroke in acute dizziness.

PITFALL 5: OVERUSE AND OVERRELIANCE ON HEAD COMPUTED TOMOGRAPHY TO RULE OUT NEUROLOGIC CAUSES

Neuroimaging can be useful in patients with acute dizziness or vertigo to diagnose (or rule out) central nervous system causes, particularly stroke, but current practice patterns do not match best evidence. In particular, there is a heavy overreliance on computed tomography (CT) of the brain,[9,41–43] despite ample evidence of its lack of utility in this clinical scenario.

The use of neuroimaging, particularly CT, has increased substantially among ED visits for dizziness over time.[9,41] In 1995, only about 10% of ED visits resulted in patients receiving a head CT scan and this increased to 25% by 2004.[9] Despite this increase in the use of neuroimaging, there was no corresponding increase over time in the proportion of patients receiving a neurologic diagnosis.[9] Contemporaneous local-area practice variation in the use of head CT by different hospitals (from 21% to 33%) does not influence the probability of identifying strokes.[43] Although CT is not recommended for diagnosis of BPPV,[6] patients diagnosed with BPPV do not have less frequent use of head CT compared with patients who receive other diagnoses.[3,4]

More recent estimates indicate that roughly 50% of ED patients with dizziness now undergo head CT.[44,45] At this frequency of use, head CT is essentially being used as a rule-out test similar to the use of cardiac enzyme biomarkers to rule out heart attack in chest pain. However, head CT is not useful to rule out stroke in acute dizziness because CT has a very low sensitivity (<40%) for acute ischemic stroke,[46] which is the most common central cause of acute dizziness presentations.[9] For posterior fossa ischemic strokes presenting dizziness, the sensitivity of CT may be even lower; it was estimated in one recent study to be just 7%.[47] Based on the low sensitivity, a negative head CT scan (the typical result in acute dizziness presentations) does not meaningfully alter the probability of acute stroke. Beyond its significant limitations as a diagnostic test, the use of head CT in dizziness presentations also has other potentially serious downsides, including an association with longer length of stay in the ED,[41] unnecessary radiation exposure, false reassurance for patients, and additional costs (hundreds of millions of dollars per year in the United States).[45]

It is sometimes suggested that CT scans are necessary to rule out brain hemorrhage. It is valid to obtain acute brain CT scans when looking for hemorrhage if a dizzy patient is hemiparetic, lethargic, or neurologically deteriorating, but screening for intracranial hemorrhage in ED patients with dizziness as the dominant symptom is highly unlikely to yield a positive result.[42] It is also reasonable to perform a CT scan to exclude brain hemorrhage if a patient is being considered for thrombolytic therapy. However, neither scenario is common, so these cannot explain the frequent use of head CT in dizziness. Instead, ingrained misconceptions,[20] medicolegal fears, patient requests, or other factors may drive neuroimaging test overuse in clinical practice.

MRI with diffusion-weighted imaging (DWI) is a more accurate test for ischemic stroke[46] and other central causes of dizziness. It is preferred to CT in clinical practice guidelines (http://www.guideline.gov/content.aspx?id=47674), and should generally be the test of choice when neuroimaging is required. However, physicians should also be cautious not to overuse MRI or overinterpret negative MRI-DWI results. MRI can substantially extend length of stay at the acute visit, and in some centers its use may require the patient to be hospitalized. Perhaps more importantly, MRI can miss acute infarction, particularly with lesions in the posterior fossa (the typical location for strokes causing dizziness or vertigo) and when it is performed within 48 hours of symptom onset.[36,48] Recent studies suggest that, in patients presenting acute, continuous dizziness, MRI-DWI misses ~10% to 20% of all strokes, including ~50% of those strokes less than 1 cm in diameter.[22,49]

SUMMARY

Opportunities exist to improve the diagnosis and management of patients with acute dizziness in routine care settings. The traditional approach to dizziness has been to determine a specific type of dizziness and then to weight this attribute heavily when formulating the case and planning further evaluation and management,[19,20] but this approach is not an evidence-based practice. Instead, providers should be focused on timing and triggers, rather than type.[28] Observational research of routine care has found that providers are frequently and increasingly using a low-value test (head CT) in typical dizziness presentations.[4,9] At the same time, providers are underusing or misusing higher-value bedside eye movement examinations.[1,4,6] To optimize the accuracy and efficiency of diagnosis in acute dizziness and vertigo, providers should deemphasize the type of dizziness, patient demographics, and the routine use of CT (or MRI) neuroimaging, and instead emphasize the timing and triggers for dizziness symptoms, leverage bedside eye movement assessments to identify opportunities to effectively and efficiently diagnose and treat common peripheral vestibular disorders, and simultaneously to determine whether MRI neuroimaging is indicated to search for dangerous central causes.

ACKNOWLEDGMENTS

Dr. Newman-Toker's effort was supported, in part, by a grant from the National Institutes of Health, National Institute on Deafness and Other Communication Disorders (1U01DC013778-01A1).

REFERENCES

1. Kerber KA, Morgenstern LB, Meurer WJ, et al. Nystagmus assessments documented by emergency physicians in acute dizziness presentations: a target for decision support? Acad Emerg Med 2011;18:619–26.
2. Royl G, Ploner CJ, Leithner C. Dizziness in the emergency room: diagnoses and misdiagnoses. Eur Neurol 2011;66:256–63.
3. Newman-Toker DE, Camargo CA Jr, Hsieh YH, et al. Disconnect between charted vestibular diagnoses and emergency department management decisions: a cross-sectional analysis from a nationally representative sample. Acad Emerg Med 2009;16:970–7.
4. Kerber KA, Burke JF, Skolarus LE, et al. Use of BPPV processes in emergency department dizziness presentations: a population-based study. Otolaryngol Head Neck Surg 2013;148:425–30.
5. von Brevern M, Radtke A, Lezius F, et al. Epidemiology of benign paroxysmal positional vertigo: a population based study. J Neurol Neurosurg Psychiatry 2007; 78:710–5.
6. Bhattacharyya N, Baugh RF, Orvidas L, et al. Clinical practice guideline: benign paroxysmal positional vertigo. Otolaryngol Head Neck Surg 2008; 139:S47–81.
7. Hilton MP, Pinder DK. The Epley (canalith repositioning) manoeuvre for benign paroxysmal positional vertigo. Cochrane Database Syst Rev 2014;(12):CD003162.
8. Hillier SL, McDonnell M. Vestibular rehabilitation for unilateral peripheral vestibular dysfunction. Cochrane Database Syst Rev 2011;(12):CD005397.
9. Kerber KA, Meurer WJ, West BT, et al. Dizziness presentations in U.S. emergency departments, 1995–2004. Acad Emerg Med 2008;15:744–50.
10. Jauch EC, Saver JL, Adams HP Jr, et al. Guidelines for the early management of patients with acute ischemic stroke: a guideline for healthcare professionals from the American Heart Association/American Stroke Association. Stroke 2013;44: 870–947.

11. Kerber KA, Brown DL, Lisabeth LD, et al. Stroke among patients with dizziness, vertigo, and imbalance in the emergency department: a population-based study. Stroke 2006;37:2484–7.
12. Newman-Toker DE, Moy E, Valente E, et al. Missed diagnosis of stroke in the emergency department: a cross-sectional analysis of a large population-based sample. Diagnosis 2014;1:155–66.
13. Paul NL, Simoni M, Rothwell PM, et al. Transient isolated brainstem symptoms preceding posterior circulation stroke: a population-based study. Lancet Neurol 2013;12:65–71.
14. Do YK, Kim J, Park CY, et al. The effect of early canalith repositioning on benign paroxysmal positional vertigo on recurrence. Clin Exp Otorhinolaryngol 2011;4: 113–7.
15. Oghalai JS, Manolidis S, Barth JL, et al. Unrecognized benign paroxysmal positional vertigo in elderly patients. Otolaryngol Head Neck Surg 2000;122:630–4.
16. Kuruvilla A, Bhattacharya P, Rajamani K, et al. Factors associated with misdiagnosis of acute stroke in young adults. J Stroke Cerebrovasc Dis 2011;20:523–7.
17. Edlow JA, Newman-Toker DE, Savitz SI. Diagnosis and initial management of cerebellar infarction. Lancet Neurol 2008;7:951–64.
18. Drachman DA, Hart CW. An approach to the dizzy patient. Neurology 1972;22: 323–34.
19. Drachman DA. A 69-year-old man with chronic dizziness. JAMA 1998;280: 2111–8.
20. Stanton VA, Hsieh YH, Camargo CA Jr, et al. Overreliance on symptom quality in diagnosing dizziness: results of a multicenter survey of emergency physicians. Mayo Clin Proc 2007;82:1319–28.
21. Newman-Toker DE, Cannon LM, Stofferahn ME, et al. Imprecision in patient reports of dizziness symptom quality: a cross-sectional study conducted in an acute care setting. Mayo Clin Proc 2007;82:1329–40.
22. Tarnutzer AA, Berkowitz AL, Robinson KA, et al. Does my dizzy patient have a stroke? A systematic review of bedside diagnosis in acute vestibular syndrome. CMAJ 2011;183:E571–92.
23. Kerber KA, Fendrick AM. The evidence base for the evaluation and management of dizziness. J Eval Clin Pract 2010;16:186–91.
24. Cheung CS, Mak PS, Manley KV, et al. Predictors of important neurological causes of dizziness among patients presenting to the emergency department. Emerg Med J 2010;27:517–21.
25. Clark MR, Sullivan MD, Fischl M, et al. Symptoms as a clue to otologic and psychiatric diagnosis in patients with dizziness. J Psychosom Res 1994;38:461–70.
26. Newman-Toker DE. Charted records of dizzy patients suggest emergency physicians emphasize symptom quality in diagnostic assessment. Ann Emerg Med 2007;50:204–5.
27. Kerber KA, Baloh RW. The evaluation of a patient with dizziness. Neurol Clin Pract 2011;1:24–33.
28. Newman-Toker DE. Symptoms and signs of neuro-otologic disorders. Continuum (Minneap Minn) 2012;18:1016–40.
29. Aw ST, Todd MJ, Aw GE, et al. Benign positional nystagmus: a study of its three-dimensional spatio-temporal characteristics. Neurology 2005;64:1897–905.
30. Neuhauser H, Leopold M, von Brevern M, et al. The interrelations of migraine, vertigo, and migrainous vertigo. Neurology 2001;56:436–41.
31. Havia M, Kentala E. Progression of symptoms of dizziness in Meniere's disease. Arch Otolaryngol Head Neck Surg 2004;130:431–5.

32. Newman-Toker DE, Stanton VA, Hsieh YH, et al. Frontline providers harbor misconceptions about the bedside evaluation of dizzy patients. Acta Otolaryngol 2008;128:601–4.
33. Baloh RW, Honrubia V, Kerber KA. Baloh and Honrubia's clinical neurophysiology of the vestibular system. 4th edition. Philadelphia: Oxford University Press; 2011.
34. Di Girolamo S, Paludetti G, Briglia G, et al. Postural control in benign paroxysmal positional vertigo before and after recovery. Acta Otolaryngol 1998;118:289–93.
35. Ruckenstein MJ. Therapeutic efficacy of the Epley canalith repositioning maneuver. Laryngoscope 2001;111:940–5.
36. Newman-Toker DE, Kerber KA, Hsieh YH, et al. HINTS outperforms ABCD2 to screen for stroke in acute continuous vertigo and dizziness. Acad Emerg Med 2013;20:986–96.
37. Hotson JR, Baloh RW. Acute vestibular syndrome. N Engl J Med 1998;339:680–5.
38. Chase M, Goldstein JN, Selim MH, et al. A prospective pilot study of predictors of acute stroke in emergency department patients with dizziness. Mayo Clin Proc 2014;89:173–80.
39. Kattah JC, Talkad AV, Wang DZ, et al. HINTS to diagnose stroke in the acute vestibular syndrome: three-step bedside oculomotor examination more sensitive than early MRI diffusion-weighted imaging. Stroke 2009;40:3504–10.
40. Martin-Schild S, Albright KC, Tanksley J, et al. Zero on the NIHSS does not equal the absence of stroke. Ann Emerg Med 2011;57:42–5.
41. Kerber KA, Schweigler L, West BT, et al. Value of computed tomography scans in ED dizziness visits: analysis from a nationally representative sample. Am J Emerg Med 2010;28:1030–6.
42. Kerber KA, Burke JF, Brown DL, et al. Does intracerebral haemorrhage mimic benign dizziness presentations? A population based study. Emerg Med J 2012;29:43–6.
43. Kim AS, Sidney S, Klingman JG, et al. Practice variation in neuroimaging to evaluate dizziness in the ED. Am J Emerg Med 2012;30(5):665–72.
44. Kerber KA, Zahuranec DB, Brown DL, et al. Stroke risk after nonstroke emergency department dizziness presentations: a population-based cohort study. Ann Neurol 2014;75:899–907.
45. Saber Tehrani AS, Coughlan D, Hsieh YH, et al. Rising annual costs of dizziness presentations to U.S. emergency departments. Acad Emerg Med 2013;20: 689–96.
46. Brazzelli M, Sandercock PA, Chappell FM, et al. Magnetic resonance imaging versus computed tomography for detection of acute vascular lesions in patients presenting with stroke symptoms. Cochrane Database Syst Rev 2009;(4):CD007424.
47. Ozono Y, Kitahara T, Fukushima M, et al. Differential diagnosis of vertigo and dizziness in the emergency department. Acta Otolaryngol 2014;134:140–5.
48. Oppenheim C, Stanescu R, Dormont D, et al. False-negative diffusion-weighted MR findings in acute ischemic stroke. AJNR Am J Neuroradiol 2000;21:1434–40.
49. Saber Tehrani AS, Kattah JC, Mantokoudis G, et al. Small strokes causing severe vertigo: frequency of false-negative MRIs and nonlacunar mechanisms. Neurology 2014;83:169–73.

TiTrATE

A Novel, Evidence-Based Approach to Diagnosing Acute Dizziness and Vertigo

David E. Newman-Toker, MD, PhD[a],*, Jonathan A. Edlow, MD[b]

KEYWORDS

- Dizziness • Vertigo • Stroke • Vestibular diseases • Diagnosis
- Medical history taking • Physical examination • Emergency departments

KEY POINTS

- The prevailing diagnostic paradigm for diagnosing emergency department (ED) patients with dizziness is based on dizziness symptom quality or type.
- Recent research suggests that the logic underlying this traditional approach is flawed.
- A newer approach based on timing and triggers of the dizziness likely offers a better diagnostic approach, especially in an unselected ED dizziness population.
- This new approach uses timing-trigger categories to define targeted bedside history and physical exam techniques to differentiate benign from dangerous causes.
- Evidence-based eye movement exams accurately discriminate BPPV (Dix-Hallpike test) and vestibular neuritis (HINTS test) from dangerous central mimics such as stroke.
- Future research should seek to prospectively study the new approach to dizziness for its overall diagnostic accuracy, resource efficiency, and impact on health outcomes.

INTRODUCTION

Dizziness accounts for 3.3% to 4.4% of ED visits.[1–3] This translates into more than 4.3 million ED patients with dizziness or vertigo annually in the United States[4] and probably 50 to 100 million worldwide.

Dizziness means different things to different people. Patients may describe feeling dizzy, lightheaded, faint, giddy, spacey, off-balance, rocking, swaying, or spinning. Expert international consensus definitions for vestibular[5] and related symptoms[6] are shown in **Box 1**. Although historically much has been made of the distinction between the terms *dizziness* and *vertigo*, current evidence (described by Kerber and Newman-Toker (Pitfalls article) elsewhere in this issue) suggests the distinction is of limited clinical usefulness. This article does not make a distinction between these terms unless specifically noted.

[a] Johns Hopkins Hospital, CRB-II, Room 2M-03 North, 1550 Orleans Street, Baltimore, MD 21231, USA; [b] Department of Emergency Medicine Administrative Offices, Beth Israel Deaconess Medical Center, West CC-2, 1 Deaconess Place, Boston, MA 02215, USA
* Corresponding author.
E-mail address: toker@jhu.edu

Neurol Clin 33 (2015) 577–599
http://dx.doi.org/10.1016/j.ncl.2015.04.011   **neurologic.theclinics.com**
0733-8619/15/$ – see front matter © 2015 Elsevier Inc. All rights reserved.

Box 1
International consensus definitions for major vestibular symptoms[5,6]

Dizziness is the sensation of disturbed or impaired spatial orientation without a false or distorted sense of motion. This includes sensations sometimes referred to as giddiness, lightheadedness, or nonspecific dizziness but does not include vertigo.

Presyncope (also near-syncope or faintness) is the sensation of impending loss of consciousness. This sensation may or may not be followed by syncope. When patients report "lightheadedness," it should be classified as presyncope, dizziness, or both.

Syncope (also faint) is transient loss of consciousness due to transient global cerebral hypoperfusion characterized by rapid onset, short duration, and spontaneous complete recovery. Syncope usually leads to loss of postural control and falling.

Vertigo is the sensation of self-motion (of head/body) when no self-motion is occurring or the sensation of distorted self-motion during an otherwise normal head movement.

Unsteadiness is the feeling of being unstable while seated, standing, or walking without a particular directional preference. This sensation has previously been called disequilibrium or imbalance.

The differential diagnosis of dizziness is broad, with no single cause accounting for more than 5% to 10% of cases.[1] This article focuses on the most common and most serious causes of new-onset dizziness in adults. More than 15% of patients presenting with dizziness to an ED have dangerous causes.[1] Sometimes, a serious cause is obvious based on the presentation (eg, dizziness with fever, cough, and hypoxia due to pneumonia). Other times, dangerous conditions can present with isolated dizziness that mimics benign problems.[7–11] Misdiagnosis in this latter group is not uncommon, even when patients are evaluated by neurologists.[12–16]

An important clinical goal is to distinguish serious from benign causes using the fewest resources possible. On average, however, diagnosing dizziness consumes disproportionate resources through extensive testing and hospital admission.[1,4] Indiscriminate application of CT, CT angiography (CTA), and MRI has low yield and low value in this patient population,[17–21] yet brain imaging for dizziness continues to increase steadily over time.[4] Use of brain imaging varies 1.5-fold across hospitals without differences in the detection of neurologic causes.[22] Annual spending on patients with dizziness in US EDs is now $4 billion,[4] with another $5 billion spent on those admitted.[23]

Previously, the evidence base for diagnosing patients with dizziness was limited.[24] A proliferation of recent research, however, has supplied clinicians with high-quality data to guide bedside diagnosis and management, particularly with regard to identifying cerebrovascular causes. This article proposes a new diagnostic paradigm based on symptom timing and triggers, derived from recent advances in evidence-based, targeted bedside examinations for specific dizziness subpopulations. New, acute dizziness presentations are focused on, and discussions about treatment are limited except where specifically relevant to initial ED management.

NEW DIAGNOSTIC APPROACH

Accumulating evidence over the past decade suggests using a different approach based on the timing and triggers for dizziness symptoms rather than type.[25,26] Timing refers to the onset, duration, and evolution of the dizziness. Triggers refer to actions, movements, or situations that provoke the onset of dizziness in patients who have intermittent symptoms.

A timing and triggers history in dizziness results in 6 possible syndromes (**Table 1**). This conceptual approach has been endorsed by an international committee of

Table 1
Timing-and-trigger–based vestibular[a] syndromes

Timing	Obligate Triggers[b] Present	No Obligate Triggers[b]
New, episodic	t-EVS (eg, BPPV)	s-EVS (eg, cardiac arrhythmia)
New, continuous	t-AVS (eg, post gentamicin)	s-AVS (eg, posterior fossa stroke)
Chronic, persistent	Context-specific chronic vestibular syndrome (eg, uncompensated unilateral vestibular loss, present only with head movement)	Spontaneous chronic vestibular syndrome (eg, chronic, persistent dizziness associated with cerebellar degeneration)

Abbreviations: t-EVS, triggered episodic vestibular syndrome; s-EVS, spontaneous episodic vestibular syndrome; t-AVS, traumatic/toxic acute vestibular syndrome; s-AVS, spontaneous acute vestibular syndrome.

[a] Note that the use of the word *vestibular* connotes vestibular symptoms (dizziness, vertigo, imbalance, or lightheadedness and so forth) rather than underlying vestibular causes (eg, BPPV or vestibular neuritis).

[b] Trigger for nonspontaneous forms refer to obligate triggers (episodic), exposures (acute, continuous), and contexts (chronic) that sharply distinguish these forms from their spontaneous counterparts. Spontaneous causes, as defined in this article, sometimes have underlying predispositions or precipitants, but these are not only-and-always associations.

Adapted from Neuro-ophthalmology Virtual Education Library. Available at: http://novel.utah. edu/newman-toker/collection.php. Accessed April 15, 2015; with permission.

specialists tasked with formulating vestibular research definitions[27] (described by Bisdorff, Staab, Newman-Toker (International Classification of Vestibular Disorders) elsewhere in this issue). Each syndrome suggests a specific differential diagnosis and targeted bedside examination, which are described further. The TiTrATE acronym stands for timing, triggers, and target examinations. The Triage–TiTrATE–Test method (**Fig. 1**) results in a new diagnostic algorithm (**Fig. 2**). This article focuses on the 4 acute

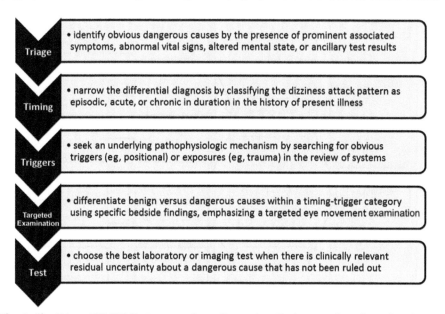

Fig. 1. The Triage–TiTrATE–Test approach to diagnosing dizziness and vertigo. The TiTrATE acronym stands for timing, triggers, and targeted examinations. (*Adapted from* Neuro-ophthalmology Virtual Education Library. Available at: http://novel.utah.edu/newman-toker/collection.php. Accessed April 15, 2015; with permission.)

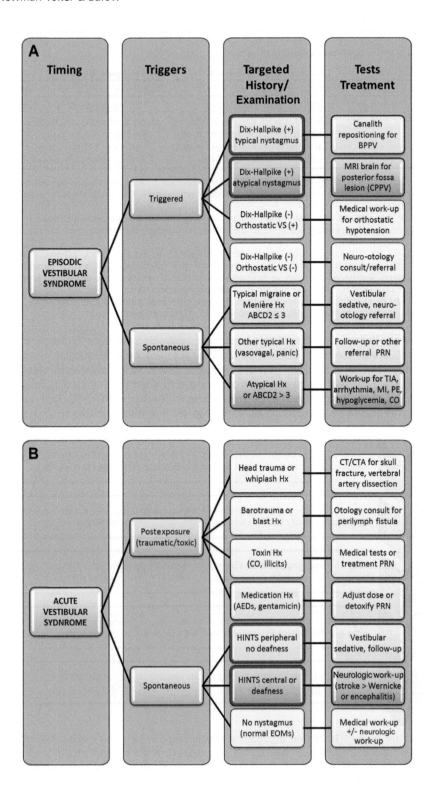

syndromes and does not discuss the 2 chronic syndromes. Some patients with a chief symptom of dizziness have prominent associated features, suggesting a likely diagnosis (**Table 2**). The emphasis is on those with isolated dizziness or vertigo. *Isolated* excludes major medical or general neurologic symptoms but includes headache and the typical otologic (eg, hearing loss, tinnitus, or ear fullness), autonomic (eg, nausea/vomiting), or balance (eg, gait unsteadiness/ataxia) accompaniments normally encountered in patients with acute vestibular symptoms.

FOUR VESTIBULAR SYNDROMES

The 4 key vestibular syndromes in ED patients presenting recent intermittent or continuous dizziness are described: triggered episodic vestibular syndrome (t-EVS), spontaneous episodic vestibular syndrome (s-EVS), traumatic/toxic acute vestibular syndrome (t-AVS), and spontaneous acute vestibular syndrome (s-AVS). The word *vestibular* refers to vestibular symptoms (dizziness, vertigo, unsteadiness, and lightheadedness), not underlying vestibular causes. For t-EVS and s-AVS, the focus is targeted bedside examination, emphasizing eye movements (**Tables 3** and **4**). For s-EVS and t-AVS, the focus is targeted history taking (see **Table 4**). Although full details for individual diseases are presented in other articles in this issue, this article summarizes key aspects related to early differential diagnostic considerations.

Episodic Vestibular Syndrome

The episodic vestibular syndrome (EVS) involves intermittent dizziness lasting seconds, minutes, or hours. Episode duration is more important than total illness duration. Most such patients have multiple, discrete episodes spaced out over time. Relapsing and remitting symptoms lasting weeks at a time, such as sometimes seen in multiple sclerosis, should not be considered in this category. EVS is divided into triggered and spontaneous forms; each is discussed.

Triggered episodic vestibular syndrome

Approach Episodes of the t-EVS are precipitated by some specific obligate action or event. The most common triggers are head motion or change in body position (eg, arising from a seated or lying position, tipping the head back in the shower to wash one's hair, or rolling over in bed). Uncommon triggers include loud sounds or Valsalva maneuvers, among others.[5] Attacks usually last seconds to minutes, depending on the underlying cause. Because some vestibular forms are provoked repetitively and

---

Fig. 2. TiTrATE algorithm for differential diagnosis and workup of dizziness and vertigo. The TiTrATE algorithm divides acute dizziness and vertigo into 4 key categories: (*A*) t-EVS and s-EVS forms of EVS and (*B*) t-AVS and s-AVS forms of AVS. Each syndrome determines a targeted bedside examination, differential diagnosis, and tests, regardless of symptom type (vertigo, presyncope, unsteadiness, or nonspecific dizziness). Some steps may occur after the ED visit, as part of follow-up or during inpatient hospital admission. Box color in the Targeted and Tests columns denotes risk of a dangerous disorder (*red*, high; *yellow*, intermediate; and *green*, low). Bold outlines denote evidence-based, targeted eye examinations that discriminate between benign and dangerous causes (see **Tables 3** and **4**). AED, antiepileptic drug; CO, carbon monoxide; EOM, extraocular movement; Hx, history; MI, myocardial infarction; PE, pulmonary embolism; PRN, pro re nata (as needed); VS, vital signs. (*Adapted from* Neuro-ophthalmology Virtual Education Library. Available at: http://novel.utah.edu/newman-toker/collection.php. Accessed April 15, 2015; with permission.)

Table 2
Prominent associated symptoms, signs, or laboratory results that may be available at the initial triage step to inform diagnosis in dizziness/vertigo

Symptom or Finding	Diagnoses That Are Suggested by the Finding
Altered mental status	Wernicke encephalopathy; stroke; encephalitis; seizure; intoxication with alcohol, illicit drugs, carbon monoxide; hypertensive encephalopathy
Transient loss of consciousness	Arrhythmia; acute coronary syndrome; aortic dissection; pulmonary embolism; vasovagal syncope; hypovolemia; stroke; subarachnoid hemorrhage; seizure
Headache	Stroke; craniocervical vascular dissection; meningitis; carbon monoxide exposure; vestibular migraine; high or low intracranial pressure; subarachnoid hemorrhage
Neck pain	Craniocervical vascular dissection (especially vertebral artery)
Chest/back pain	Acute coronary syndrome; aortic dissection
Abdominal/back pain	Ruptured ectopic pregnancy; aortic dissection
Dyspnea	Pulmonary embolism; pneumonia; anemia
Palpitations	Arrhythmia; vasovagal syncope; panic disorder
Bleeding or fluid losses	Hypovolemia; anemia
New/recent medication use	Medication side effects or toxicity (eg, gentamicin)
Fever or chills	Systemic infection; encephalitis; mastoiditis; meningitis
Abnormal glucose	Symptomatic hypoglycemia; diabetic ketoacidosis

frequently or patients' nausea can linger between spells, some patients may overstate episode duration. This can usually be sorted out by careful history taking.

It bears emphasis that clinicians must distinguish triggers (head or body motion provokes new symptoms not present at baseline) from exacerbating features (head or body motion worsens preexisting baseline dizziness). Head movement typically exacerbates any dizziness of vestibular cause (benign or dangerous, central or peripheral, or acute or chronic). The concept that worsening of dizziness with head motion equates with a peripheral cause is a common misconception.[28]

The goal of physical examination in t-EVS is to reproduce a patient's dizziness to witness the corresponding pathophysiology (eg, falling blood pressure on arising or abnormal eye movements with Dix-Hallpike testing). A caveat for postural symptoms is that orthostatic dizziness and orthostatic hypotension are not always related.[29,30] Orthostatic hypotension may be incidental and misleading, especially in older patients taking antihypertensive medications.[31] Conversely, dizziness on arising without systemic orthostatic hypotension may indicate hemodynamic transient ischemic attack (TIA) from hypoperfusion distal to a cranial vascular stenosis[32] or, alternatively, intracranial hypotension.[33] Neurologic evaluation is probably indicated for patients with reproducible and sustained orthostatic dizziness but no demonstrable hypotension or benign paroxysmal positional vertigo (BPPV).

Prototype t-EVS causes are BPPV and orthostatic hypotension. Dangerous causes include neurologic mimics, known as central paroxysmal positional vertigo (CPPV) (eg, posterior fossa mass lesions[34]), and serious causes of orthostatic hypotension,[35] such as internal bleeding. All are associated with episodic positional symptoms but can be readily distinguished from one another using targeted bedside history and examination. Orthostatic hypotension causes symptoms only on arising, whereas BPPV causes symptoms both on arising and on lying back or when rolling in bed.[36] BPPV

Table 3
Nystagmus characteristics in key peripheral and central vestibular disorders

Vestibular Condition	Test Maneuver	Nystagmus Duration	Trajectory/Direction	Variation in Direction
t-EVS[a] (episodic nystagmus triggered by specific positional maneuvers)				
Posterior canal BPPV	Head hanging with 45° turn to each side (Dix-Hallpike test)	5–30 s[b]	*Upbeat-torsional*[c]	Direction reversal on arising
Horizontal canal BPPV	Supine roll to either side (Pagnini–McClure maneuver)	30–90 s[b]	Horizontal	*Spontaneous reversal during test*
CPPV	Any (usually head hanging)	5–60+ s[b] (sometimes **persistent** if position is held)	Any (usually **downbeat** or horizontal)	Any (often direction fixed)
s-AVS[a] (spontaneous nystagmus that may be exacerbated nonspecifically by various head maneuvers)				
Vestibular neuritis or labyrinthitis	Gaze testing[d]	Persistent	Dominantly horizontal	Direction fixed (acutely)
Stroke	Gaze testing[d]	Persistent	Any (usually dominantly horizontal, occasionally **vertical or torsional**)	Direction fixed or **direction changing** with gaze position

Italic: very likely peripheral nystagmus; Bold: very likely central nystagmus; Roman: indeterminate nystagmus (other eye movement features may be diagnostic).

[a] Only 2 syndromes (t-EVS and s-AVS) are shown in this table because the other 2 syndromes (s-EVS and t-AVS) lack characteristic, diagnostic patterns of nystagmus.

[b] BPPV nystagmus usually begins after a delay (latency) of a few seconds, peaks in intensity rapidly, then decays in intensity rapidly, peaks in intensity rapidly, then decays in intensity rapidly, then decays in intensity rapidly, then decays in intensity rapidly. In the horizontal canal variant, the nystagmus may be biphasic, with a spontaneous direction reversal after the initial nystagmus, even if the head is held motionless. CPPV may begin immediately or after a delay, may decay or persist, and may or may not change direction during testing.

[c] Torsion with the 12-o'clock pole (top) of the eye beating toward down-facing (tested) ear, sometimes referred to as geotropic (ie, toward the ground).

[d] In the AVS, gaze testing is useful but positional tests are not. With peripheral lesions, nystagmus should increase in intensity when a patient's gaze is directed toward the fast phase of the nystagmus and should not reverse. With central lesions, this same pattern may occur, but more than one-third of the time, the nystagmus reverses direction when the patient's gaze is directed away from the fast phase of the nystagmus (ie, is direction changing with gaze position).

Adapted from Neuro-ophthalmology Virtual Education Library. Available at: http://novel.utah.edu/newman-toker/collection.php. Accessed April 15, 2015; with permission.

Table 4
Safe-to-go features for the most common, benign vestibular[a] causes of isolated dizziness and vertigo

Syndrome[b]	Targeted Examination	Benign Disorder	Dangerous Mimic	Safe-to-Go Features
t-EVS	Orthostatic vitals; positional tests for nystagmus	BPPV	Posterior fossa mass	• No pain, auditory, neurologic symptoms, or syncope • Symptoms not limited to arising and occur when tipping head forward/back or rolling in bed • Asymptomatic with head stationary, symptoms reproduced by specific positional tests (see **Table 3**) • Characteristic, canal-specific, peripheral-type nystagmus on positional tests (see **Table 3**) • Therapeutic response to canal-specific repositioning maneuvers (posterior canal: modified Epley maneuver; horizontal canal: Lempert roll [barbecue] maneuver)[40]
s-EVS	Head, neck, and cranial nerve history; ear, hearing history	Vestibular migraine or Menière disease	TIA	• No cardiorespiratory symptoms or transient loss of consciousness • No diplopia or other dangerous D symptoms (dysarthria, dysphagia, dysphonia, dysmetria)[96] • No papilledema, Horner syndrome, cranial nerve signs (eg, facial palsy, especially if headache present • No sudden, severe, or sustained pain (especially located in the posterior neck) • Strong/long past history of dizziness episodes (at least 5 spells over >2 years) • Clear precipitants (eg, stress, food, visual motion) for multiple episodes or ABCD[2] risk score ≤3 • Migraine: history of migraine headache; classic visual aura or photophobia with most attacks • Menière: history of unilateral fluctuating hearing loss or tinnitus with most attacks

| s-AVS | HINTS; ear, hearing examination | Vestibular neuritis | Stroke[c] |

Stroke[c] findings:

- Maximum 1 prodromal spell <48 h before onset
- No excessive vomiting or gait disorder
- No pain, auditory, neurologic symptoms
- No papilledema, Horner syndrome, cranial nerve signs (eg, facial palsy), especially if headache present
- Stands and walks unassisted (even if unsteady or wide based, unable to perform tandem gait)
- HINTS plus hearing/ear examination—SEND HIM ON HOME[96]:
  o SEND—straight eyes (no vertical ocular misalignment, also known as skew), no deafness
  o HIM—head impulse misses (unilateral abnormal impulse opposite nystagmus direction)
  o ON—one-way nystagmus (unidirectional nystagmus worse in gaze toward fast phase)
  o HOME—healthy otic and mastoid examination (pearly tympanic membrane with no pimples, pus, or perforation; no pain on palpation of the mastoid)

[a] Vestibular disorders are highlighted because ED physicians have a high degree of comfort diagnosing other benign causes of isolated t-EVS (eg, orthostatic hypotension) and isolated s-EVS (eg, vasovagal syncope). Dangerous nonvestibular, non-neurologic causes (principally for s-EVS) are rarely isolated (see **Table 2**).

[b] Only 3 syndromes (t-EVS, s-EVS, and s-AVS) are shown in this table because the other syndrome (t-AVS) is typically diagnosed largely on exposure history. Findings on the HINTS examination that suggest stroke are given the acronym INFARCT (impulse normal, fast-phase alternating, and refixation on cover test).[96] Thus, if an s-AVS patient has any 1 of these 3 eye signs (bilaterally normal head impulses; direction-changing, gaze-evoked nystagmus; or vertical skew deviation), stroke is likely.

[c] *Adapted from* Neuro-ophthalmology Virtual Education Library. Available at: http://novel.utah.edu/newman-toker/collection.php. Accessed April 15, 2015; with permission.

and CPPV can be distinguished based on characteristic eye examination differences on standard positional tests for nystagmus, including the Dix-Hallpike test (see **Table 3**).[37]

Diseases BPPV is the most common vestibular disorder in the general population, with a lifetime prevalence of 2.4% and increasing incidence with age.[36] In the ED, it is probably the second most common cause, accounting for approximately 10% of ED dizzy presentations.[16] It results from mobile crystalline debris trapped in 1 or more semicircular canals (canaliths) within the vestibular labyrinth. Symptoms and signs vary based on the canal(s) involved and whether the crystals are free-floating or trapped.[38] Classic symptoms are repetitive, brief, triggered episodes of rotational vertigo lasting more than a few seconds but less than 1 minute, although nonvertiginous symptoms of dizziness or even presyncope is frequent.[39]

The diagnosis is confirmed by reproducing symptoms and signs using canal-specific positional testing maneuvers and identifying a canal-specific nystagmus (see **Table 3**).[38] Because the offending canal(s) are generally not known in advance, multiple diagnostic maneuvers are typically performed. Proven bedside treatments to displace the offending crystals (canalith repositioning maneuvers) are also canal specific.[37,40] As discussed previously, BPPV mimics include orthostatic hypotension and CPPV. Patients with atypical nystagmus forms (eg, downbeat or horizontal) on Dix-Hallpike testing usually have CPPV, and some cases are due to posterior fossa tumors or strokes.[37] CPPV includes common, benign causes, such as intoxication with alcohol or sedative drugs, but such patients are more apt to complain of continuous, persistent dizziness exacerbated (rather than triggered) by position change and are usually readily diagnosed based on context and other signs of intoxication.

Orthostatic hypotension is common, accounting for 24% of acute syncopal spells.[41] Classic symptoms are brief lightheadedness or a feeling of near-syncope on arising, but vertigo is common[42] and underappreciated.[28] Orthostatic hypotension is caused by numerous conditions that produce hypovolemia, cardiac dysfunction, or reduced vasomotor tone. The most common causes are medications and hypovolemia.[41]

The primary dangerous concern is internal bleeding. Strong bedside predictors of moderate hypovolemia from blood loss are postural dizziness so severe as to prevent standing and a postural pulse increment greater than 30 beats per minute, but the sensitivity of these findings is only 22%.[43] Furthermore, the benign postural orthostatic tachycardia syndrome produces similar clinical findings.[6] Heart rate is not a consistent predictor of serious disease; absence of tachycardia or even relative bradycardia can occur in catastrophic conditions, such as ruptured ectopic pregnancy. Coexistent chest, back, abdominal, or pelvic pain should suggest intrathoracic or intra-abdominal emergencies. Dangerous diseases presenting severe orthostatic hypotension but sometimes lacking overt clues include myocardial infarction, occult sepsis, adrenal insufficiency, and diabetic ketoacidosis.[35]

Spontaneous episodic vestibular syndrome
Approach Episode duration for s-EVS varies, ranging from seconds to a few days, but a majority of spells last minutes to hours.[44] Patients are often asymptomatic at the time of ED presentation. Because episodes cannot usually be provoked at the bedside (as they can with the t-EVS), evaluation relies almost entirely on history taking. The frequency of spells varies from multiple times a day to monthly, depending on the cause. Although precipitants may exist (eg, red wine prior to vestibular migraine), many spells occur without apparent provocation. This differs from BPPV and other diseases with obligate, immediate triggers. Diagnosis may be clear-cut in typical

cases. Unfortunately, classic features, such as frank loss of consciousness in vaso-vagal syncope,[45] headache in vestibular migraine,[46] and fear in panic attacks,[47] are absent in 25% to 35% of cases. Atypical case presentations probably contribute to diagnostic confusion in patients with such transient neurologic attacks.[48]

Prototype s-EVS causes include common benign, recurrent disorders, such as vestibular migraine, vasovagal syncope, and panic attacks. Although Ménière disease is often mentioned as a common cause of s-EVS, its estimated population prevalence (0.1%[49]) is much lower than that of the 3 other episodic disorders. Principal dangerous causes are cerebrovascular (vertebrobasilar TIA and subarachnoid hemorrhage), cardiorespiratory (cardiac arrhythmia, unstable angina, and pulmonary embolus), and endocrine (hypoglycemia). Temporary or intermittent carbon monoxide exposure is a rare serious cause.[50]

Diseases Patients with Ménière disease classically present with episodic vertigo accompanied by unilateral tinnitus and aural fullness, often with reversible sensori-neural hearing loss.[51] Only 1 in 4 initially presents with the complete symptom triad,[52] and nonvertiginous dizziness is common.[53] Patients with suspected Ménière disease should generally be referred to an otolaryngologist, but care must be taken to avoid missing TIA mimics with audiovestibular symptoms.[54]

Vestibular migraine (previously called migrainous vertigo, migraine-associated vertigo, or migraine-associated dizziness) is a newly described form of migraine. It is related to basilar-type migraine,[55] but episodes lack a second defining brainstem symptom, such as diplopia, quadriparesis, or paresthesias.[56] The 2 migraine types may exist along a continuum.[57] With a population prevalence of approximately 1%,[58] vestibular migraine is a common cause of s-EVS. A definite diagnosis of vesti-bular migraine requires greater than or equal to 5 attacks with vestibular symptoms, a history of migraine headaches, and migraine-like symptoms with at least half the at-tacks.[59] Episode duration ranges from seconds to days.[56] Nystagmus, if present, may be peripheral, central, or mixed-type.[56] Headache is often absent.[46] When head-ache does occur, it may begin before, during, or after the dizziness and may differ from the patient's other typical migraine headaches.[56] Nausea, vomiting, photophobia, phonophobia, and visual auras may occur. There are no pathognomonic signs or bio-markers, so diagnosis is currently based on clinical history and exclusion of alternative causes.[59] An episode similar to prior spells with long illness duration, migraine features, no red flags, and low vascular risk is sufficient for diagnosis without testing (see **Table 4**).

Reflex syncope (also called neurocardiogenic or neurally mediated syncope) usually has prodromal symptoms, typically lasting 3 to 30 minutes.[60] Dizziness, the most common prodrome, occurs in 70% to 75%[61–63] and may be of any type, including vertigo.[61] Although rarely seen in clinical practice, central forms of nystagmus may be identified during provocative testing, suggesting a TIA-like mechanism producing central vertigo.[64] In reflex syncope, episodes of near-syncope (no loss of conscious-ness) substantially outnumber spells with syncope,[63] so many patients likely present with isolated dizziness. The diagnosis is readily suspected if classic contextual precip-itants (eg, pain/fear for vasovagal syncope and micturition/defecation for situational syncope) are present,[65] but these are absent in atypical forms, including those due to carotid sinus hypersensitivity.[6] Diagnosis is based on clinical history, excluding dangerous mimics (especially cardiac arrhythmia), and, if clinically necessary, can be confirmed by formal head-up tilt table testing.[6]

Panic attacks, with or without hyperventilation, are often accompanied by episodic dizziness. Dizziness begins rapidly, peaks within 10 minutes and, by definition, is accompanied by at least 3 other symptoms.[66] There may be a situational precipitant (eg, claustrophobia), but spells often occur spontaneously. Fear of dying or going crazy are classic symptoms but are absent in 30% of cases.[47] Ictal panic attacks from temporal lobe epilepsy generally last only seconds, and altered mental status is frequent.[67] Hypoglycemia, cardiac arrhythmias, pheochromocytoma, and basilar TIA can all mimic panic attacks presenting with dizziness; each can produce a multi-symptom complex with neurologic and autonomic features.

The most common dangerous diagnoses for s-EVS are TIA and cardiac arrhythmias. In 1975, a National Institutes of Health consensus report on TIA recommended that isolated dizziness or vertigo not be considered a TIA,[68] a pronouncement that has been widely accepted. Recent data, however, contradict this classic teaching. Multiple studies show that dizziness and vertigo, even when isolated, are the most common premonitory vertebrobasilar TIA symptoms and are more frequent in the days to weeks preceding posterior circulation stroke.[69–71]

TIAs can present with isolated episodes of dizziness weeks to months prior to a completed infarction.[72,73] Dizziness is the most common presenting symptom of vertebral artery dissection,[74] which affects younger patients, mimics migraine, and is easily misdiagnosed.[13] Dizziness and vertigo are the most common symptoms in basilar artery occlusion and are sometimes early and isolated.[75,76] Because approximately 5% of TIA patients suffer a stroke within 48 hours[77] and rapid treatment reduces stroke risk by up to 80%,[78,79] prompt diagnosis is critical. Patients with posterior circulation TIA have an even higher stroke risk than those with anterior circulation spells.[80,81] The presence of 3 or more vascular risk factors or an ABCD^2 score greater than or equal to 4 is a predictor of TIA in patients with s-EVS,[82,83] although high-risk vascular lesions may predict stroke risk more accurately than risk factor–based scoring.[84]

Cardiac arrhythmias should be considered in any patient with s-EVS, particularly when syncope occurs or when exertion is a precipitant, even if the lead symptom is true spinning vertigo.[10,42] Although some clinical features during the attack may increase or decrease the odds of a dangerous cardiac cause,[65] additional testing (eg, cardiac loop recording) is often required to confirm the final diagnosis.[6]

Acute Vestibular Syndrome

The acute vestibular syndrome (AVS) involves acute, persistent dizziness lasting days to weeks, sometimes with lingering sequelae thereafter. Temporal evolution at onset and in the first week is more important than total illness duration. Most such patients have a monophasic course with an early peak in symptom severity, rapid improvement in symptoms over the first week, and gradual recovery over weeks to months. Unusual cases resolve in less than 48 to 72 hours. AVS is divided into postexposure (traumatic/toxic) and spontaneous forms; each is discussed.

Traumatic/toxic acute vestibular syndrome
Approach Sometimes AVS results directly from trauma or a toxic exposure (t-AVS). The exposure history is usually obvious. The most common causes are blunt head injury and drug intoxication, particularly with medications (eg, anticonvulsants) or illicit substances affecting the brainstem, cerebellum, or peripheral vestibular apparatus.

Most patients experience a single, acute attack resolving gradually over days to weeks once the exposure has stopped. Depending on the nature of the trauma or toxin, other symptoms, such as headache or altered mental status, may predominate. Rotatory vertigo, spontaneous nystagmus (looking straight ahead), and head-motion intolerance may be absent or unimpressive if the pathologic effects are bilateral and relatively symmetric, as with most toxins.

Diseases Blunt head trauma,[85] blast injuries,[86] whiplash,[87] and barotrauma[88] may cause direct vestibular nerve injury, labyrinthine concussion, or mechanical disruption of inner ear membranes, resulting in an AVS presentation. Care should be taken not to miss a basal skull fracture or traumatic vertebral artery dissection. Traumatic brain injury may cause the postconcussion syndrome. Patients typically present with a combination of dizziness, headaches, fatigue, and minor cognitive impairments, with dizziness the most common symptom in the first 2 weeks after injury.[89]

Anticonvulsant side effects or toxicity is a frequent cause of dizziness and vertigo in the ED and may present with an acute clinical picture.[90] Carbon monoxide intoxication is an uncommon but important cause to consider.[91] Aminoglycoside toxicity is a well-known cause of acute bilateral vestibular failure.[92,93] Gentamicin produces profound, permanent loss of vestibular function with relatively spared hearing, and toxicity may occur after even a single antibiotic dose.[93] Although this problem is often discovered during the course of an inpatient admission, patients may develop symptoms later and present to the ED. Patients usually present with predominantly gait unsteadiness and oscillopsia (bouncing vision) while walking.[94]

Spontaneous acute vestibular syndrome

Approach Classic AVS is defined as the acute onset of persistent, continuous dizziness or vertigo in association with nausea or vomiting, gait instability, nystagmus, and head-motion intolerance that lasts days to weeks.[95] Patients are usually symptomatic at the time of ED presentation and focused physical examination is usually diagnostic. Patients generally experience worsening of AVS symptoms with any head motion, including provocative tests (eg, Dix-Hallpike test). Contrary to conventional wisdom, these exacerbating features do not suggest an etiologic or anatomic diagnosis[95] and must be distinguished from head movements that trigger dizziness.[96] This common source of confusion probably contributes to misdiagnosis of a peripheral problem or positional vertigo when dizziness worsens with head movement or testing.[28,97] The difference is that a patient with s-AVS is dizzy at rest and feels worse with any head motion, whereas a patient with t-EVS is normal at rest and specific head motions induce transient dizziness. This means that positional tests, such as Dix-Hallpike test, should not be applied to AVS patients but reserved for use in EVS.

The prototype s-AVS cause is vestibular neuritis (often incorrectly called labyrinthitis), an acute peripheral vestibulopathy without hearing loss. The primary dangerous mimic is ischemic stroke in the lateral brainstem, cerebellum, or inner ear.[95] Cerebellar hemorrhages rarely mimic a peripheral vestibular process.[98] Uncommon dangerous causes are thiamine deficiency[11] and listeria encephalitis.[99]

Although it is often assumed that strokes usually exhibit neurologic features,[28] obvious focal signs are present in fewer than 20% of stroke patients with s-AVS.[95] Patients are usually symptomatic at initial assessment and often have diagnostic eye signs. Strong evidence[95] suggests that a physical examination clinical decision rule using 3 bedside eye examination findings (HINTS—head impulse test, nystagmus type, and skew deviation; see **Table 4**) rules out stroke more accurately than early MRI.[90,100,101] Importantly, the mere presence of nystagmus (found in both neuritis and stroke) is not as useful as the nystagmus attributes, which help differentiate the 2 (see **Table 3**).

Eye movement tests have excellent performance characteristics in the hands of neuro-otologists, and similar findings have been replicated by multiple investigative teams around the world.[102–107] Nevertheless, care should be taken before applying these tests in routine ED practice, because interpretation differs between experts and novices[108] and limited instruction may not always be sufficient to yield optimal results.[16] More extensive training with subspecialists directly observing trainees and providing immediate feedback may facilitate skill-building at tertiary care institutions with access to such expertise,[109] but new technologies may offer more widely available help in the near future. Recent studies have found accurate diagnosis using a portable video-oculography device that measures key eye movements quantitatively.[110,111] Such devices could eventually make subspecialty-level expertise in eye movement assessment widely available for diagnosis or training, although artifacts and related issues with quantitative recordings still currently require expert interpretation.[112]

Neuroimaging studies are often insufficient to accurately diagnose s-AVS cases. CT, the most commonly applied test, is useful to detect (or rule out) brain hemorrhages but is far less helpful for investigating suspected ischemic strokes. Retrospective studies suggest CT may have up to 42% sensitivity for ischemic stroke in dizziness.[19,113] In prospective studies, however, CT has even lower sensitivity (16%) for detecting early acute ischemic stroke,[114] especially in the posterior fossa (7%).[107] CT should, therefore, not be used to exclude ischemic stroke in s-AVS.[115] Lack of understanding of CT's limitations for assessment of dizziness may lead to CT overuse and misdiagnosis.[13,28] Less well known is that even MRI with diffusion-weighted imaging (DWI) misses 10% to 20% of strokes in s-AVS during the first 24 to 48 hours.[95,101] When smaller strokes (<1 cm in diameter) present with s-AVS, early MRI sensitivity is only approximately 50%.[116] Repeat delayed MRI-DWI (3–7 days after onset of symptoms) may be required to confirm a new infarct.[90,117] Routine MRI in all ED dizziness also has a low yield.[21] Imaging only older patients with vascular risk factors is a common practice, but the countervailing concern is that young age predisposes to missed stroke.[13,118,119] Stroke risk in patients presenting isolated s-AVS and no vascular risk factors is still approximately 10% to 20%, and 1 in 4 strokes occurs in a patient under age 50.[95] Overreliance on youth, low vascular risk, normal neurologic examination, and normal CT likely explains the high odds of missed stroke in isolated dizziness, particularly among younger stroke victims.[12,14,120]

Diseases Vestibular neuritis is a benign, self-limited condition affecting the vestibular nerve. Some cases are linked to specific causes (eg, multiple sclerosis[121]), but most are idiopathic and possibly related to herpes simplex infections.[122] Although vestibular neuritis is usually a monophasic illness, 25% of cases have a single brief prodrome in the week prior to the attack[123] and others have recurrences months or years later.[124] MRI with or without contrast is normal and unnecessary.[125] Diagnosis is based on nystagmus type and vestibular reflexes.[126] Early treatment with oral or intravenous steroids is supported by some evidence but remains controversial.[127]

When hearing loss accompanies vertigo in a neuritis-like s-AVS presentation, the syndrome is known as viral labyrinthitis, although cochleovestibular neuritis might be more appropriate. This benign presentation must be differentiated from bacterial labyrinthitis, a dangerous disorder resulting from spread of middle ear or systemic infection that may lead to meningitis if left untreated.[128] Even in the absence of systemic or local (otitis or mastoiditis) infection, however, this presentation should be viewed suspiciously, because inner ear strokes typically present this way[54,106,129] and may often be the cause of s-AVS with hearing loss in the ED.[101]

The prevalence of stroke in ED dizziness is 3% to 5%[1,2,12,16,130,131] and probably less for those with isolated dizziness.[12] Among ED dizzy patients, those with AVS are a high-risk subgroup for stroke (approximately 25% of s-AVS cases).[95] Posterior circulation stroke typically presents with s-AVS, sometimes after a series of sponta-neous episodes in the preceding weeks or months (ie, TIAs, usually from posterior circulation stenosis, culminating in stroke).[95] Almost all of these strokes (96%) are ischemic.[95,98] Most are initially associated with minor neurologic disability that re-covers well, absent recurrent stroke. Delays in prompt diagnosis and treatment, how-ever, can result in serious permanent disability or death.[13,95] Although most such patients are not thrombolysis candidates by current guidelines, they may benefit from early secondary prevention treatments and interventions to prevent posterior fossa stroke complications.[95,115]

BEDSIDE APPROACH SUMMARY

For the usual ED patient with isolated dizziness or vertigo that is not obviously of traumatic or toxic cause, the goal for the syndrome-specific targeted examination is to firmly diagnose the specific benign conditions described previously. A majority of cases with initial diagnostic uncertainty are due to common cardiovascular (medica-tion-induced orthostatic hypotension and vasovagal syncope), psychiatric (panic dis-order), or vestibular (BPPV, vestibular migraine, and vestibular neuritis) disorders. These benign conditions can each be diagnosed confidently at the bedside using a syndrome-targeted history and examination. Patients whose presentations are atypical or whose targeted examination findings are suspicious for dangerous under-lying causes should undergo appropriate laboratory tests, imaging, or consultation.

Bedside examinations for benign vestibular disorders probably deserve special attention in emergency medicine education and in developing decision support tools.[114,128,129] Confusion over the conduct of these examinations may stem from the fact that a given clinical feature (eg, upbeat-torsional nystagmus) predicts a benign condition in one syndrome (t-EVS, indicating typical posterior-canal BPPV) but a dangerous one in another (s-AVS, indicating a brainstem stroke).[28] Thus, it is crucial to identify the timing-and-trigger syndrome before targeting the examination, some-thing seldom done in current practice, and, unfortunately, often omitted in prominent textbooks[132–134] and journal articles.[135] Key criteria that define typical benign vesti-bular disorder cases and differentiate them from dangerous neurologic causes are shown in **Tables 3** and **4**.

SUMMARY

The prevailing diagnostic paradigm for diagnosing ED patients with dizziness is based on dizziness symptom quality or type. Recent research suggests that the logic under-lying this traditional approach is flawed. A newer approach based on timing and triggers of the dizziness likely offers a better diagnostic approach, especially in an un-selected ED dizziness population. Using this approach allows targeted bedside exam-inations of proven value to be used effectively. Future research should seek to prospectively study the new approach to dizziness for its overall diagnostic accuracy, resource efficiency, and impact on health outcomes.

ACKNOWLEDGMENTS

Dr. Newman-Toker's effort was supported, in part, by a grant from the National Institutes of Health, National Institute on Deafness and Other Communication Disor-ders (1U01DC013778-01A1).

APPENDIX

In the spirit of the flipped classroom, the guest editors of this *Neurologic Clinics of North America* issue on "Emergency Neuro-Otology: Diagnosis and Management of Acute Dizziness and Vertigo" have assembled a collection of unknown cases to be accessed electronically in multimedia format. By design, cases are not linked with specific articles, to avoid untoward cueing effects for the learner. The cases are real and are meant to demonstrate and reinforce lessons provided in this and subsequent articles. In addition to pertinent elements of medical history, cases include videos of key examination findings.

A hyperlink to a URL is provided for a secure server that houses the 10 cases. Note that additional cases may be added over time. Simply click on a case you wish to view and advance at your leisure. The purpose of the cases is illustrative, and there are no quizzes. Please click on this link to be directed to the interactive cases:

https://connect.johnshopkins.edu/vertigooverview/

The authors hope you enjoy the final result.

REFERENCES

1. Newman-Toker DE, Hsieh YH, Camargo CA Jr, et al. Spectrum of dizziness visits to US emergency departments: cross-sectional analysis from a nationally representative sample. Mayo Clin Proc 2008;83(7):765–75.
2. Cheung CS, Mak PS, Manley KV, et al. Predictors of important neurological causes of dizziness among patients presenting to the emergency department. Emerg Med J 2010;27(7):517–21.
3. Newman-Toker DE, Cannon LM, Stofferahn ME, et al. Imprecision in patient reports of dizziness symptom quality: a cross-sectional study conducted in an acute care setting. Mayo Clin Proc 2007;82(11):1329–40.
4. Saber Tehrani AS, Coughlan D, Hsieh YH, et al. Rising annual costs of dizziness presentations to u.s. Emergency departments. Acad Emerg Med 2013;20(7):689–96.
5. Bisdorff A, Von Brevern M, Lempert T, et al. Classification of vestibular symptoms: towards an international classification of vestibular disorders. J Vestib Res 2009;19(1–2):1–13.
6. Moya A, Sutton R, Ammirati F, et al. Guidelines for the diagnosis and management of syncope (version 2009). Eur Heart J 2009;30(21):2631–71.
7. Malouf R, Brust JC. Hypoglycemia: causes, neurological manifestations, and outcome. Ann Neurol 1985;17(5):421–30.
8. Lee H, Sohn SI, Cho YW, et al. Cerebellar infarction presenting isolated vertigo: frequency and vascular topographical patterns. Neurology 2006;67(7):1178–83.
9. Demiryoguran NS, Karcioglu O, Topacoglu H, et al. Painless aortic dissection with bilateral carotid involvement presenting with vertigo as the chief complaint. Emerg Med J 2006;23(2):e15.
10. Newman-Toker DE, Camargo CA Jr. 'Cardiogenic vertigo'–true vertigo as the presenting manifestation of primary cardiac disease. Nat Clin Pract Neurol 2006;2(3):167–72 [quiz: 173].
11. Kattah JC, Dhanani SD, Pula JH, et al. Vestibular signs of thiamine deficiency during the early phase of suspected Wernicke's encephalopathy. Neurol Clin Pract 2013;3:460–8.
12. Kerber KA, Brown DL, Lisabeth LD, et al. Stroke among patients with dizziness, vertigo, and imbalance in the emergency department: a population-based study. Stroke 2006;37(10):2484–7.

13. Savitz SI, Caplan LR, Edlow JA. Pitfalls in the diagnosis of cerebellar infarction. Acad Emerg Med 2007;14(1):63–8.
14. Kim AS, Fullerton HJ, Johnston SC. Risk of vascular events in emergency department patients discharged home with diagnosis of dizziness or vertigo. Ann Emerg Med 2011;57(1):34–41.
15. Braun EM, Tomazic PV, Ropposch T, et al. Misdiagnosis of acute peripheral vestibulopathy in central nervous ischemic infarction. Otol Neurotol 2011;32(9): 1518–21.
16. Royl G, Ploner CJ, Leithner C. Dizziness in the emergency room: diagnoses and misdiagnoses. Eur Neurol 2011;66(5):256–63.
17. Wasay M, Dubey N, Bakshi R. Dizziness and yield of emergency head CT scan: is it cost effective? Emerg Med J 2005;22(4):312.
18. Kerber KA, Schweigler L, West BT, et al. Value of computed tomography scans in ED dizziness visits: analysis from a nationally representative sample. Am J Emerg Med 2010;28(9):1030–6.
19. Lawhn-Heath C, Buckle C, Christoforidis G, et al. Utility of head CT in the evaluation of vertigo/dizziness in the emergency department. Emerg Radiol 2013;20(1):45–9.
20. Fakhran S, Alhilali L, Branstetter BF 4th. Yield of CT angiography and contrast-enhanced MR imaging in patients with dizziness. AJNR Am J Neuroradiol 2013; 34(5):1077–81.
21. Ahsan SF, Syamal MN, Yaremchuk K, et al. The costs and utility of imaging in evaluating dizzy patients in the emergency room. Laryngoscope 2013;123(9): 2250–3.
22. Kim AS, Sidney S, Klingman JG, et al. Practice variation in neuroimaging to evaluate dizziness in the ED. Am J Emerg Med 2012;30(5):665–72.
23. Newman-Toker DE, McDonald KM, Meltzer DO. How much diagnostic safety can we afford, and how should we decide? A health economics perspective. BMJ Qual Saf 2013;22(Suppl 2):ii11–20.
24. Kerber KA, Fendrick AM. The evidence base for the evaluation and management of dizziness. J Eval Clin Pract 2010;16(1):186–91.
25. Newman-Toker DE. Diagnosing dizziness in the emergency department-why "what do you mean by 'dizzy'?" Should not be the first question you ask. Baltimore (MD): The Johns Hopkins University; 2007 [Doctoral Dissertation, Clinical Investigation, Bloomberg School of Public Health]. ProQuest Digital Dissertations [database on Internet]; publication number: AAT 3267879. Available at: http://www.proquest.com/ http://gateway.proquest.com/openurl?url_ver=Z39. 88-2004&res_dat=xri:pqdiss&rft_val_fmt=info:ofi/fmt:kev:mtx:dissertation&rft_ dat=xri:pqdiss:3267879. Accessed April 15, 2015.
26. Edlow JA. Diagnosing dizziness: we are teaching the wrong paradigm! Acad Emerg Med 2013;20(10):1064–6.
27. Newman-Toker DE, Staab JP, Bronstein A, et al. Proposed multi-layer structure for the international classification of vestibular disorders [abstract]. Bárány Society XXVI International Congress. Reykjavik, Iceland, August 18–21, 2010.
28. Stanton VA, Hsieh YH, Camargo CA Jr, et al. Overreliance on symptom quality in diagnosing dizziness: results of a multicenter survey of emergency physicians. Mayo Clin Proc 2007;82(11):1319–28.
29. Radtke A, Lempert T, von Brevern M, et al. Prevalence and complications of orthostatic dizziness in the general population. Clin Auton Res 2011;21(3):161–8.
30. Wu JS, Yang YC, Lu FH, et al. Population-based study on the prevalence and correlates of orthostatic hypotension/hypertension and orthostatic dizziness. Hypertens Res 2008;31(5):897–904.

31. Poon IO, Braun U. High prevalence of orthostatic hypotension and its correlation with potentially causative medications among elderly veterans. J Clin Pharm Ther 2005;30(2):173–8.

32. Stark RJ, Wodak J. Primary orthostatic cerebral ischaemia. J Neurol Neurosurg Psychiatry 1983;46(10):883–91.

33. Blank SC, Shakir RA, Bindoff LA, et al. Spontaneous intracranial hypotension: clinical and magnetic resonance imaging characteristics. Clin Neurol Neurosurg 1997;99(3):199–204.

34. Buttner U, Helmchen C, Brandt T. Diagnostic criteria for central versus peripheral positioning nystagmus and vertigo: a review. Acta Otolaryngol 1999;119(1):1–5.

35. Gilbert VE. Immediate orthostatic hypotension: diagnostic value in acutely ill patients. South Med J 1993;86(9):1028–32.

36. von Brevern M, Radtke A, Lezius F, et al. Epidemiology of benign paroxysmal positional vertigo: a population based study. J Neurol Neurosurg Psychiatry 2007;78(7):710–5.

37. Bhattacharyya N, Baugh RF, Orvidas L, et al. Clinical practice guideline: benign paroxysmal positional vertigo. Otolaryngol Head Neck Surg 2008;139(5 Suppl 4):S47–81.

38. von Brevern M, Bertholon P, Brandt T, et al. Benign paroxysmal positional vertigo: diagnostic criteria. J Vestib Res, in press.

39. Lawson J, Johnson I, Bamiou DE, et al. Benign paroxysmal positional vertigo: clinical characteristics of dizzy patients referred to a Falls and Syncope Unit. QJM 2005;98(5):357–64.

40. Fife TD, Iverson DJ, Lempert T, et al. Practice parameter: therapies for benign paroxysmal positional vertigo (an evidence-based review): report of the Quality Standards Subcommittee of the American Academy of Neurology. Neurology 2008;70(22):2067–74.

41. Sarasin FP, Louis-Simonet M, Carballo D, et al. Prevalence of orthostatic hypotension among patients presenting with syncope in the ED. Am J Emerg Med 2002;20(6):497–501.

42. Newman-Toker DE, Dy FJ, Stanton VA, et al. How often is dizziness from primary cardiovascular disease true vertigo? A systematic review. J Gen Intern Med 2008;23(12):2087–94.

43. McGee S, Abernethy WB 3rd, Simel DL. The rational clinical examination. Is this patient hypovolemic? JAMA 1999;281(11):1022–9.

44. Lempert T. Recurrent spontaneous attacks of dizziness. Continuum 2012;18(5 Neuro-otology):1086–101.

45. Mathias CJ, Deguchi K, Schatz I. Observations on recurrent syncope and presyncope in 641 patients. Lancet 2001;357(9253):348–53.

46. Dieterich M, Brandt T. Episodic vertigo related to migraine (90 cases): vestibular migraine? J Neurol 1999;246(10):883–92.

47. Chen J, Tsuchiya M, Kawakami N, et al. Non-fearful vs. fearful panic attacks: a general population study from the National Comorbidity Survey. J Affect Disord 2009;112(1–3):273–8.

48. Fonseca AC, Canhao P. Diagnostic difficulties in the classification of transient neurological attacks. Eur J Neurol 2011;18:644–8.

49. Radtke A, von Brevern M, Feldmann M, et al. Screening for Meniere's disease in the general population - the needle in the haystack. Acta Otolaryngol 2008;128(3):272–6.

50. Keles A, Demircan A, Kurtoglu G. Carbon monoxide poisoning: how many patients do we miss? Eur J Emerg Med 2008;15(3):154–7.

51. Sajjadi H, Paparella MM. Meniere's disease. Lancet 2008;372(9636):406–14.
52. Mancini F, Catalani M, Carru M, et al. History of Meniere's disease and its clinical presentation. Otolaryngol Clin North Am 2002;35(3):565–80.
53. Faag C, Bergenius J, Forsberg C, et al. Symptoms experienced by patients with peripheral vestibular disorders: evaluation of the Vertigo Symptom Scale for clinical application. Clin Otolaryngol 2007;32(6):440–6.
54. Lee H. Audiovestibular loss in anterior inferior cerebellar artery territory infarction: a window to early detection? J Neurol Sci 2012;313(1–2):153–9.
55. Kirchmann M, Thomsen LL, Olesen J. Basilar-type migraine: clinical, epidemiologic, and genetic features. Neurology 2006;66(6):880–6.
56. Lempert T, Neuhauser H, Daroff RB. Vertigo as a symptom of migraine. Ann N Y Acad Sci 2009;1164:242–51.
57. Wang CT, Lai MS, Young YH. Relationship between basilar-type migraine and migrainous vertigo. Headache 2009;49(3):426–34.
58. Neuhauser HK, Radtke A, von Brevern M, et al. Migrainous vertigo: prevalence and impact on quality of life. Neurology 2006;67(6):1028–33.
59. Lempert T, Olesen J, Furman J, et al. Vestibular migraine: diagnostic criteria. J Vestib Res 2012;22(4):167–72.
60. Sheldon RS, Amuah JE, Connolly SJ, et al. Design and use of a quantitative scale for measuring presyncope. J Cardiovasc Electrophysiol 2009;20(8):888–93.
61. Sloane PD, Linzer M, Pontinen M, et al. Clinical significance of a dizziness history in medical patients with syncope. Arch Intern Med 1991;151(8):1625–8.
62. Calkins H, Shyr Y, Frumin H, et al. The value of the clinical history in the differentiation of syncope due to ventricular tachycardia, atrioventricular block, and neurocardiogenic syncope. Am J Med 1995;98(4):365–73.
63. Romme JJ, van Dijk N, Boer KR, et al. Influence of age and gender on the occurrence and presentation of reflex syncope. Clin Auton Res 2008;18(3):127–33.
64. Choi JH, Seo JD, Kim MJ, et al. Vertigo and nystagmus in orthostatic hypotension. Eur J Neurol 2015;22(4):648–55.
65. van Dijk JG, Thijs RD, Benditt DG, et al. A guide to disorders causing transient loss of consciousness: focus on syncope. Nat Rev Neurol 2009;5(8):438–48.
66. Katon WJ. Clinical practice. Panic disorder. N Engl J Med 2006;354(22):2360–7.
67. Kanner AM. Ictal panic and interictal panic attacks: diagnostic and therapeutic principles. Neurol Clin 2011;29(1):163–75, ix.
68. A classification and outline of cerebrovascular diseases. II. Stroke 1975;6(5):564–616.
69. Compter A, Kappelle LJ, Algra A, et al. Nonfocal symptoms are more frequent in patients with vertebral artery than carotid artery stenosis. Cerebrovasc Dis 2013;35(4):378–84.
70. Hoshino T, Nagao T, Mizuno S, et al. Transient neurological attack before vertebrobasilar stroke. J Neurol Sci 2013;325(1–2):39–42.
71. Paul NL, Simoni M, Rothwell PM, et al. Transient isolated brainstem symptoms preceding posterior circulation stroke: a population-based study. Lancet Neurol 2013;12(1):65–71.
72. Grad A, Baloh RW. Vertigo of vascular origin. Clinical and electronystagmographic features in 84 cases. Arch Neurol 1989;46(3):281–4.
73. Gomez CR, Cruz-Flores S, Malkoff MD, et al. Isolated vertigo as a manifestation of vertebrobasilar ischemia. Neurology 1996;47(1):94–7.
74. Gottesman RF, Sharma P, Robinson KA, et al. Clinical characteristics of symptomatic vertebral artery dissection: a systematic review. Neurologist 2012;18(5):245–54.

75. Fisher CM. Vertigo in cerebrovascular disease. Arch Otolaryngol 1967;85(5): 529–34.
76. von Campe G, Regli F, Bogousslavsky J. Heralding manifestations of basilar artery occlusion with lethal or severe stroke. J Neurol Neurosurg Psychiatry 2003; 74(12):1621–6.
77. Shah KH, Kleckner K, Edlow JA. Short-term prognosis of stroke among patients diagnosed in the emergency department with a transient ischemic attack. Ann Emerg Med 2008;51(3):316–23.
78. Lavallee PC, Meseguer E, Abboud H, et al. A transient ischaemic attack clinic with round-the-clock access (SOS-TIA): feasibility and effects. Lancet Neurol 2007;6(11):953–60.
79. Rothwell PM, Giles MF, Chandratheva A, et al. Effect of urgent treatment of transient ischaemic attack and minor stroke on early recurrent stroke (EXPRESS study): a prospective population-based sequential comparison. Lancet 2007; 370(9596):1432–42.
80. Flossmann E, Rothwell PM. Prognosis of vertebrobasilar transient ischaemic attack and minor stroke. Brain 2003;126(Pt 9):1940–54.
81. Gulli G, Khan S, Markus HS. Vertebrobasilar stenosis predicts high early recurrent stroke risk in posterior circulation stroke and TIA. Stroke 2009;40(8):2732–7.
82. Moubayed SP, Saliba I. Vertebrobasilar insufficiency presenting as isolated positional vertigo or dizziness: a double-blind retrospective cohort study. Laryngoscope 2009;119(10):2071–6.
83. Navi BB, Kamel H, Shah MP, et al. Application of the ABCD2 score to identify cerebrovascular causes of dizziness in the emergency department. Stroke 2012;43(6):1484–9.
84. Amarenco P, Labreuche J, Lavallee PC. Patients with transient ischemic attack with ABCD2 <4 can have similar 90-day stroke risk as patients with transient ischemic attack with ABCD2 ≥4. Stroke 2012;43(3):863–5.
85. Davies RA, Luxon LM. Dizziness following head injury: a neuro-otological study. J Neurol 1995;242(4):222–30.
86. Hoffer ME, Balaban C, Gottshall K, et al. Blast exposure: vestibular consequences and associated characteristics. Otol Neurotol 2010;31(2):232–6.
87. Vibert D, Hausler R. Acute peripheral vestibular deficits after whiplash injuries. Ann Otol Rhinol Laryngol 2003;112(3):246–51.
88. Klingmann C, Praetorius M, Baumann I, et al. Barotrauma and decompression illness of the inner ear: 46 cases during treatment and follow-up. Otol Neurotol 2007;28(4):447–54.
89. Yang CC, Tu YK, Hua MS, et al. The association between the postconcussion symptoms and clinical outcomes for patients with mild traumatic brain injury. J Trauma 2007;62(3):657–63.
90. Kattah JC, Talkad AV, Wang DZ, et al. HINTS to diagnose stroke in the acute vestibular syndrome: three-step bedside oculomotor examination more sensitive than early MRI diffusion-weighted imaging. Stroke 2009;40(11):3504–10.
91. Trevino R. A 19-year-old woman with unexplained weakness and dizziness. J Emerg Nurs 1997;23(5):499–500.
92. Ariano RE, Zelenitsky SA, Kassum DA. Aminoglycoside-induced vestibular injury: maintaining a sense of balance. Ann Pharmacother 2008;42(9):1282–9.
93. Ahmed RM, Hannigan IP, MacDougall HG, et al. Gentamicin ototoxicity: a 23-year selected case series of 103 patients. Med J Aust 2012;196(11):701–4.
94. Crawford J. Living without a balancing mechanism. N Engl J Med 1952;246(12): 458–60.

95. Tarnutzer AA, Berkowitz AL, Robinson KA, et al. Does my dizzy patient have a stroke? A systematic review of bedside diagnosis in acute vestibular syndrome. CMAJ 2011;183(9):E571–592.

96. Newman-Toker DE. Symptoms and signs of neuro-otologic disorders. Continuum (Minneap Minn) 2012;18(5 Neuro-otology):1016–40.

97. Newman-Toker DE, Stanton VA, Hsieh YH, et al. Frontline providers harbor misconceptions about the bedside evaluation of dizzy patients. Acta Otolaryngol 2008;128(5):601–4.

98. Kerber KA, Burke JF, Brown DL, et al. Does intracerebral haemorrhage mimic benign dizziness presentations? A population based study. Emerg Med J 2012;29(1):43–6.

99. Smiatacz T, Kowalik MM, Hlebowicz M. Prolonged dysphagia due to Listeria-rhombencephalitis with brainstem abscess and acute polyradiculoneuritis. J Infect 2006;52(6):e165–7.

100. Newman-Toker DE, Kattah JC, Alvernia JE, et al. Normal head impulse test differentiates acute cerebellar strokes from vestibular neuritis. Neurology 2008;70(24 Pt 2):2378–85.

101. Newman-Toker DE, Kerber KA, Hsieh YH, et al. HINTS Outperforms ABCD2 to screen for stroke in acute continuous vertigo and dizziness. Acad Emerg Med 2013;20(10):986–96.

102. Cnyrim CD, Newman-Toker D, Karch C, et al. Bedside differentiation of vestibular neuritis from central "vestibular pseudoneuritis". J Neurol Neurosurg Psychiatry 2008;79(4):458–60.

103. Chen L, Lee W, Chambers BR, et al. Diagnostic accuracy of acute vestibular syndrome at the bedside in a stroke unit. J Neurol 2011;258(5):855–61.

104. Casani AP, Dallan I, Cerchiai N, et al. Cerebellar infarctions mimicking acute peripheral vertigo: how to avoid misdiagnosis? Otolaryngol Head Neck Surg 2013;148(3):475–81.

105. Kim MB, Boo SH, Ban JH. Nystagmus-based approach to vertebrobasilar stroke presenting as vertigo without initial neurologic signs. Eur Neurol 2013;70(5–6):322–8.

106. Huh YE, Koo JW, Lee H, et al. Head-Shaking aids in the diagnosis of acute audiovestibular loss due to anterior inferior cerebellar artery infarction. Audiol Neurootol 2013;18(2):114–24.

107. Ozono Y, Kitahara T, Fukushima M, et al. Differential diagnosis of vertigo and dizziness in the emergency department. Acta Otolaryngol 2014;134(2):140–5.

108. Jorns-Haderli M, Straumann D, Palla A. Accuracy of the bedside head impulse test in detecting vestibular hypofunction. J Neurol Neurosurg Psychiatry 2007;78(10):1113–8.

109. Vanni S, Nazerian P, Casati C, et al. Can emergency physicians accurately and reliably assess acute vertigo in the emergency department? Emerg Med Australas 2015;27(2):126–31.

110. Newman-Toker DE, Saber Tehrani AS, Mantokoudis G, et al. Quantitative videooculography to help diagnose stroke in acute vertigo and dizziness: toward an ECG for the eyes. Stroke 2013;44(4):1158–61.

111. Mantokoudis G, Tehrani AS, Wozniak A, et al. VOR gain by head impulse videooculography differentiates acute vestibular neuritis from stroke. Otol Neurotol 2015;36(3):457–65.

112. Mantokoudis G, Saber Tehrani AS, Kattah JC, et al. Quantifying the vestibulo-ocular reflex with video-oculography: nature and frequency of artifacts. Audiol Neurootol 2015;20(1):39–50.

113. Hwang DY, Silva GS, Furie KL, et al. Comparative sensitivity of computed tomography vs. magnetic resonance imaging for detecting acute posterior fossa infarct. J Emerg Med 2012;42(5):559–65.

114. Chalela JA, Kidwell CS, Nentwich LM, et al. Magnetic resonance imaging and computed tomography in emergency assessment of patients with suspected acute stroke: a prospective comparison. Lancet 2007;369(9558):293–8.

115. Edlow JA, Newman-Toker DE, Savitz SI. Diagnosis and initial management of cerebellar infarction. Lancet Neurol 2008;7(10):951–64.

116. Saber Tehrani AS, Kattah JC, Mantokoudis G, et al. Small strokes causing severe vertigo: frequency of false-negative MRIs and nonlacunar mechanisms. Neurology 2014;83(2):169–73.

117. Morita S, Suzuki M, Iizuka K. False-negative diffusion-weighted MRI in acute cerebellar stroke. Auris Nasus Larynx 2011;38(5):577–82.

118. Bhattacharya P, Nagaraja N, Rajamani K, et al. Early use of MRI improves diagnostic accuracy in young adults with stroke. J Neurol Sci 2013;324(1–2):62–4.

119. Newman-Toker DE, Moy E, Valente E, et al. Missed diagnosis of stroke in the emergency department: a cross-sectional analysis of a large population-based sample. Diagnosis 2014;1(2):155–66.

120. Lee CC, Ho HC, Su YC, et al. Increased risk of vascular events in emergency room patients discharged home with diagnosis of dizziness or vertigo: a 3-year follow-up study. PLoS One 2012;7(4):e35923.

121. Pula JH, Newman-Toker DE, Kattah JC. Multiple sclerosis as a cause of the acute vestibular syndrome. J Neurol 2013;260(6):1649–54.

122. Arbusow V, Theil D, Strupp M, et al. HSV-1 not only in human vestibular ganglia but also in the vestibular labyrinth. Audiol Neurootol 2001;6(5):259–62.

123. Lee H, Kim BK, Park HJ, et al. Prodromal dizziness in vestibular neuritis: frequency and clinical implication. J Neurol Neurosurg Psychiatry 2009;80(3):355–6.

124. Bergenius J, Perols O. Vestibular neuritis: a follow-up study. Acta Otolaryngol 1999;119(8):895–9.

125. Strupp M, Jager L, Muller-Lisse U, et al. High resolution Gd-DTPA MR imaging of the inner ear in 60 patients with idiopathic vestibular neuritis: no evidence for contrast enhancement of the labyrinth or vestibular nerve. J Vestib Res 1998; 8(6):427–33.

126. Kim JS, Kim HJ. Inferior vestibular neuritis. J Neurol 2012;259(8):1553–60.

127. Wegner I, van Benthem PP, Aarts MC, et al. Insufficient evidence for the effect of corticosteroid treatment on recovery of vestibular neuritis. Otolaryngol Head Neck Surg 2012;147(5):826–31.

128. Bergmann K. Fatal complications of otitis 60 years ago. HNO 1995;43(8):478–81 [in German].

129. Kim JS, Cho KH, Lee H. Isolated labyrinthine infarction as a harbinger of anterior inferior cerebellar artery territory infarction with normal diffusion-weighted brain MRI. J Neurol Sci 2009;278(1–2):82–4.

130. Navi BB, Kamel H, Shah MP, et al. Rate and predictors of serious neurologic causes of dizziness in the emergency department. Mayo Clin Proc 2012; 87(11):1080–8.

131. Lee DH, Kim WY, Shim BS, et al. Characteristics of central lesions in patients with dizziness determined by diffusion MRI in the emergency department. Emerg Med J 2014;31(8):641–4.

132. Raynor EM. Vertigo. In: Wolfson AB, Hendey GW, Ling LJ, et al, editors. Harwood-nuss' clinical practice of emergency medicine. 5th edition. Philadelphia: Lippincott Williams & Wilkins; 2010.

133. Goldman B. Vertigo and dizziness. In: Tintinalli JE, Stapczynski JS, Ma OJ, et al, editors. Emergency medicine: a comprehensive study guide. 7th edition. New York: McGraw-Hill, Medical Pub. Division; 2011.

134. Chang AK, Olshaker JS. Dizziness and Vertigo. In: Marx JA, Hockberger RS, Walls RM, editors. Rosen's emergency medicine concepts and clinical practice. 8th edition. Philadelphia: Saunders/Elsevier; 2014. p. 162–169.e1.

135. Ning M, Gonzalez RG. Case records of the Massachusetts General Hospital. Case 34-2013. A 69-year-old man with dizziness and vomiting. N Engl J Med 2013;369(18):1736–48.

Section II – Acute, Episodic Dizziness and Vertigo

Benign Paroxysmal Positional Vertigo in the Acute Care Setting

Terry D. Fife, MD[a],*, Michael von Brevern, MD[b]

KEYWORDS

- Dizziness • Positional vertigo • Paroxysmal vertigo
- Canalith repositioning maneuver • Liberatory maneuver • Canalolithiasis
- Cupulolithiasis

KEY POINTS

- Benign paroxysmal positional vertigo (BPPV) is a common cause of vertigo caused by calcium carbonate sediment originating from the utricle that dislodges and falls into one of the semicircular canals.
- BPPV usually causes brief attacks of spinning vertigo (10–20 seconds) induced by head position changes.
- Dix Hallpike positioning toward the affected side in posterior canal BPPV is associated with a 1- to 10-second latency and a fast phase.
- Treatment is achieved by "repositioning" calcium carbonate sediment from the posterior semicircular canal to the main vestibule.
- Treatment of posterior canal BPPV using the canalith repositioning maneuvers is effective in more than 90% of patients.

CASE SCENARIO

A 62-year-old woman presents to the emergency department reporting severe dizziness that came on abruptly at 4 AM. She recalls getting up from bed and felt "thrown" back to the bed and could barely stagger to the bathroom. She recalls having intense vertigo and feels unsteady on her feet when she tries to walk. She does not recall any prior similar vertigo and has not had slurred speech, diplopia, limb clumsiness, headache, or hearing loss. On physical examination, she can cautiously get up from bed but feels more "woozy" in doing so. There are no focal examination deficits, but Dix

Disclosures: Dr M. von Brevern has nothing to disclose; Dr T.D. Fife has nothing to disclose.
[a] Department of Neurology, Barrow Neurological Institute, University of Arizona College of Medicine, 240 West Thomas Road, Suite 301, Phoenix, AZ 85013, USA; [b] Department of Neurology, Park-Klinik Weissensee, Schoenstrasse 80, Berlin 13086, Germany
* Corresponding author.
E-mail address: tfife@email.arizona.edu

Neurol Clin 33 (2015) 601–617
http://dx.doi.org/10.1016/j.ncl.2015.04.003   neurologic.theclinics.com
0733-8619/15/$ – see front matter © 2015 Elsevier Inc. All rights reserved.

Hallpike positioning to the right side results in pronounced paroxysmal positional nystagmus.

EPIDEMIOLOGY

Benign paroxysmal positional vertigo (BPPV) is the most common cause of vertigo and its incidence increases with advancing age.[1] Unrecognized BPPV can be found in about 10% of certain geriatric populations[2,3] and there is a cumulative incidence of nearly 10% by age 80.[4] BPPV has a lifetime prevalence of 3.2% in women, 1.6% in men, and an overall prevalence of 2.4% in the adult general population.[4]

BPPV may be associated with trauma or viral infection, but the majority of cases are idiopathic.[5] BPPV is the most common vestibular problem, following head trauma.[6] About 13% of traumatic brain injury patients complain of positional vertigo and one-half have BPPV responsive to treatment.[7] BPPV owing to trauma is usually apparent within 1 week of head trauma as long as the patient has been moving sufficiently to provoke symptoms.[8] Adding to the challenge of diagnosis, acute vestibular neuritis can be associated with BPPV, possibly owing to inflammatory effects in the labyrinth or by affecting labyrinthine perfusion.[9] Idiopathic BPPV is about twice as common among women compared with men, whereas BPPV associated with trauma or viral neurolabyrinthitis occur with about equal frequency across genders.[5]

PATHOPHYSIOLOGY

BPPV is caused by calcium carbonate debris that erodes or becomes dislodged from the macula within the utricle. The calcium carbonate material has a density of 2.7 g/mL, which is considerably greater than that of endolymph (about 1 g/mL), so it moves or "sinks" by the effect of gravity and may fall into one of the semicircular canals.[10] The posterior canal is positioned anatomically to be the most likely recipient, which is why close to 80% of BPPV is related to the posterior canal. The term "canalolithiasis" refers to the most common mechanism of BPPV, in which mobile calcium debris triggers abnormal activation of the ampullary nerve. The term "cupulolithiasis" refers to the less common mechanism in which the calcium material is stuck to the cupula itself, causing inappropriate ampullary nerve activation.[11] The cupula is the gel-like structure in the ampulla of each semicircular canal that transduces mechanical endolymph flow into electrochemical nerve signals allowing the central nervous system to sense acceleration in the plane of that canal. This mechanism is supported by the response to canalith repositioning maneuvers, animal models,[12,13] abnormal utricular function in BPPV as determined by ocular vestibular evoked myogenic potential studies,[14] and a mathematical analysis.[15]

The calcium carbonate material seems to originate from the otoconia of the macule of the utricle. It is not well-understood why the material dislodges, but studies in aging rats showed pitting, fissuring, and cracking of otoconia and disruption of linking filaments, all of which correlated with advancing age.[16] Similar age-related changes have been demonstrated by scanning electron microscopy in specimens from the otoconia from the utricles of 5 humans, ranging in age from 47 to 63 years.[17] Osteoporosis and osteopenia may be factors increasing the likelihood of erosion and degeneration of otoconia.[18] Such a process could potentially explain the greater prevalence of idiopathic BPPV in women because of estrogen effects on calcium deposition. The number of otoconia and size was diminished in osteoporotic rats.[19] Postmenopausal women with BPPV had a high prevalence of osteopenia and osteoporosis.[20] Genetic factors leading to predisposition for BPPV may also prove important in some patients; 1 large family suggested linkage to a region on chromosome 15.[21]

DIAGNOSIS

The most typical presentation is of a patient greater than 20 years old reporting recurrent sensations of spinning with turning in bed or tilting the head. Many but not all patients have discovered the association between head movements and the onset of vertigo, and some have developed strategies to avoid provoking the attacks by sleeping while sitting up or taking care to move slowly. Spells are brief, usually less than 30 seconds, and are unaccompanied by changes in hearing or focal neurologic signs. Some patients develop mild dizziness or unsteadiness between spells owing possibly to very mild BPPV symptoms or owing to other mechanisms. Although the history is characteristic, some well-intentioned patients do not relay a history of positional vertigo or of recurrent brief attacks. Examination with Dix Hallpike maneuver can be helpful in recognizing such otherwise unexplained dizziness particularly in older patients.[3,12] Because it can be difficult to reliably distinguish the variant of BPPV by canal type base only on history, the diagnosis and feature of the nystagmus related to each canal are discussed elsewhere in this article.

Each of the 3 semicircular canals of the labyrinth may be affected by canalolithiasis or cupulolithiasis. Because the opening of the posterior canal is in the dependent position when we are flat, it is predisposed anatomically to receive calcium debris more often. Hence the posterior canal form of BPPV accounts for about 80% to 90% of cases. About 15% of BPPV is related to the horizontal canal. It is estimated that about 1% to 2% of BPPV may be related to the anterior canal, which is mostly seen in the course of the calcium debris moving from 1 canal to another during repositioning maneuvers. When the calcium material changes from 1 canal to another, it is sometimes referred to as "canal switch."[22] Involvement of more than 1 canal at a time is another condition encountered in some patients.[23–25] Bilateral BPPV is seen particularly in traumatic BPPV.[26,27]

Treating BPPV owing to canalolithiasis is accomplished by moving otolithic material from the lumen of the affected semicircular canal back in to the utricle where it came from. Meanwhile, BPPV owing to cupulolithiasis is best achieved by maneuvers that cause the otolithic material to dislodge from the cupula, so that it moves freely and can respond to maneuvers that move it back in to the utricle once again.

Posterior Canal Benign Paroxysmal Positional Vertigo

Diagnosis

The nystagmus that is characteristic of the posterior canal form of BPPV can be induced by the Dix Hallpike maneuver (**Fig. 1**) or by the so-called side-lying maneuver (**Fig. 2**). Once the patient's head has come to rest in the dependent position, after a brief latency of a few seconds, the nystagmus begins if the ear that is down is affected by BPPV. The nystagmus is a combination of upbeating and cyclotorsional nystagmus with the top pole of the rotational component beating toward the side of the down ear (**Table 1**). Recall that the nystagmus direction is defined by the direction of the fast phase because it is the easiest to observe. Observing nystagmus with these directional features that comes on after a brief latency and lasts fewer than 30 seconds, which correlates with the patient's sensation of dizziness, ascertains the diagnosis to the posterior canal on side with the lower ear.

Treatment

There are 2 established, safe, and effective maneuvers to treat posterior canal BPPV[28–31] (1): the canalith (or canalolith) repositioning procedure, also known as the

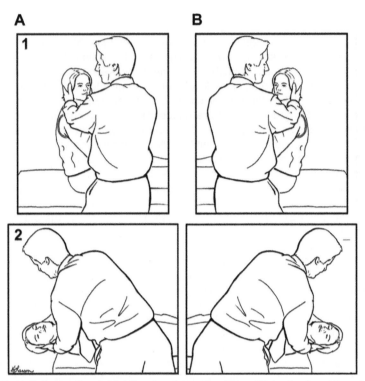

Fig. 1. Dix Hallpike to the right (*A*) going from the sitting (1) to the head hanging right position (2). Dix Hallpike to the left (*B*).

Epley maneuver (**Fig. 3**), and (2) the liberatory maneuver, also known as the Semont maneuver (**Fig. 4**).[32] The initial step of each therapeutic maneuver is identical to a diagnostic procedure. The first steps of the canalith repositioning procedure comprise the Dix Hallpike maneuver so that the therapeutic maneuver can be done by proceeding from the Dix Hallpike maneuver if nystagmus is seen. Similarly, the first step of the

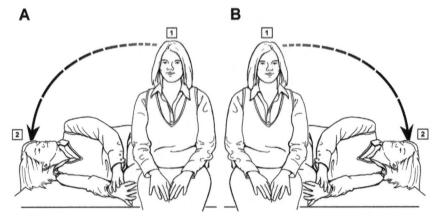

Fig. 2. The side-lying maneuver for posterior canal benign paroxysmal positional vertigo on the right (*A*) and left (*B*) sides. Number 1 represents the initial upright position and 2 represents the position to which the patient is moved on each respective side.

Table 1
Direction of paroxysmal positional nystagmus by benign paroxysmal positional vertigo (BPPV) canal type

BPPV Canal Involved	Direction of Paroxysmal Nystagmus (Direction of the Fast Phase)
Posterior canal BPPV (tested by Dix Hallpike maneuver; see **Fig. 1**)	Upbeating and torsional with the top pole of rotation beating toward the lower ear
Horizontal canal BPPV (tested by supine roll test; see **Fig. 3**)	Geotropic type (presumed canalolithiasis): Geotropic direction changing horizontal nystagmus (ie, paroxysmal right beating with supine head turn to the right and left beating with supine head turn to the left Apogeotropic type (presumed cupulolithiasis): Apogeotropic direction changing horizontal nystagmus (ie, paroxysmal right beating with supine head turn to the left and left beating with supine head turn to the right)
Anterior canal BPPV (test by straight head hanging or Dix Hallpike maneuver)	Downbeating, with a minor torsional component

Semont maneuver constitutes the side-lying test, and treatment may proceed directly from the side-lying maneuver.

A number of modifications of these maneuvers have been devised and may very well work, but with 2 proven effective maneuvers that are easy to perform, there is usually no need to find other, equally effective maneuvers. When patients do not respond, it may be owing to the technique and particularly owing to insufficient head extension during the Epley maneuver. The other cause can simply be a refractory case and in those cases surgical canal plugging can be considered. There is no clear consensus on how many times to do the maneuver to perform at a single visit, but the authors' preference is 2 or 3 times if nystagmus is still present with the second maneuver.

What if the history suggests BPPV but Dix Hallpike positioning provokes transient vertigo without visible nystagmus? In these cases, it is reasonable to treat the patient anyway.[12,33,34] The absence of nystagmus may be owing to insufficient calcium movement to stimulate the ampulla. High-resolution MRI of the membranous labyrinth seemed to show irregularities in the lumen with regions of narrowing or stenosis, which might affect the free movement of otolithic material preventing the inducement of nystagmus and potentially also making treatment less effective.[35] In addition, some patients actually do have resolution of BPPV but report persisting dizziness. Some such cases may be owing to anxiety and a sense of fear that they might develop the vertigo.[36] Persisting dizziness may improve with reassurance and patient education.[37]

Posttreatment instructions
There are few scientific data on whether posttreatment instructions affect outcome. A recent metaanalysis concluded that postural restrictions for 1 to several days after successful treatment of BPPV of the posterior canal (including avoidance of laying on the affected ear and sleeping upright) slightly reduce the recurrence rate.[38] However, these restrictions are unpleasant for patients and not recommended by many experts. Pretreatment with vestibular suppressant medications is not needed in most cases, but may help to improve patient comfort for those particularly susceptible to motion sickness.

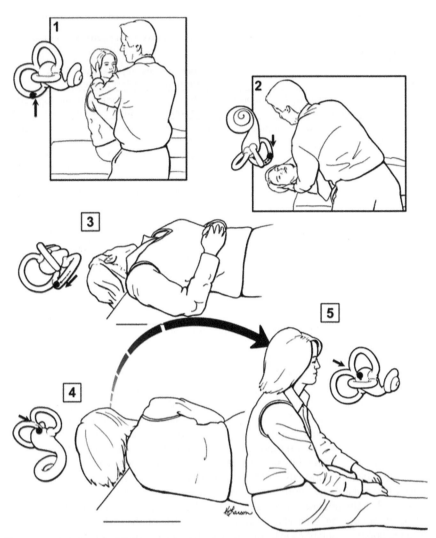

Fig. 3. Canalith (Canalolith) Repositioning Maneuver for Right Side. Steps: [1] Have the patient sit on a table positioned so that he or she may be laid back to the head-hanging position with the neck in slight extension. Stabilize the head and move it 45 degrees toward the side to be tested. [2] Move the head, neck, and shoulders all together to avoid neck strain. Observe the eyes for nystagmus; hold them open, if necessary. If nystagmus is seen, wait for all nystagmus to abate and hold the position another 15 seconds. [3] While the head is slightly hyperextended, turn the head 90 degrees toward the opposite side, and wait 30 seconds. [4] Roll the body to the the lateral body position, turn the patient's head toward the ground so that the patient is facing straight down and hold for 15 seconds. [5] While maintaining the head position unchanged relative to the shoulders, have the patient sit up and hold on to the patient for 5 seconds or so to guard against momentary dizziness upon sitting up. This maneuver may be repeated several times or until symptoms and nystagmus cannot be reproduced.

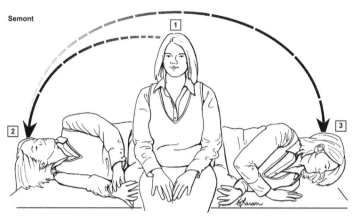

Fig. 4. Semont's Liberatory Maneuver for Treatment of Right BPPV. Steps in performing Semont's liberatory maneuver: [1] with the patient on a table or flat surface, turn the head away from the affected side (assuming it is known). [2] Rapidly move the patient to the side-lying position, toward the affected side with the head turned 45 degrees up. Nystagmus will be seen at this point if the patient has BPPV of the posterior canal on that side. Hold the patient there for 30 seconds or until all nystagmus has stopped. [3] Rapidly move the patient to the opposite side position with the head facing 45 degrees down (the head should not change position relative to the shoulder during this step) and hold there for 30 seconds. Finally, bring the patient back up from position [3] back to the sitting position.

Home self-treatment for benign paroxysmal positional vertigo

Many patients can complete these treatment maneuvers successfully at home, or at least try treating themselves first before returning to a physician or therapist for treatment.[39] Radtke and colleagues[40] found that patients who self-treated using the Semont liberatory experienced resolution of vertigo and nystagmus 58% of the time and those self-treating with canalith repositioning (Epley) maneuver had 95% resolution after 1 week. Still, not all patients are capable of performing these maneuvers on their own for various reasons. There is substantial interest from the lay public in how to self-manage and treat their own dizziness and Youtube.com and other web-based information is sought frequently by the public.[41,42]

Horizontal Canal Benign Paroxysmal Positional Vertigo

Diagnosis

Although the nystagmus of horizontal canal BPPV might sometimes be provoked by the Dix Hallpike maneuver, the supine roll test (**Fig. 5**) is a more effective test of its presence.[12,43,44] The nystagmus of horizontal canal BPPV is different from that of posterior canal BPPV (see **Table 1**). Horizontal canal BPPV is associated with horizontal direction changing positional nystagmus. There are 2 types of direction-changing positional nystagmus that might be seen. The first and most common form is geotropic (toward the earth) and probably caused by canalolithiasis.[45] That is, from the supine position when the head is turned to the right, the nystagmus is right beating and when it is turned to the left it changes to become left beating.[46] The second, less common, and somewhat less responsive to treatment is the apogeotropic (away from earth) type, which is often owing to cupulolithiasis. For testing of the horizontal canal, the head of the patient in the supine position is elevated about 30° and then turned quickly to either side (see **Fig. 5**). The resulting nystagmus usually has a short latency,

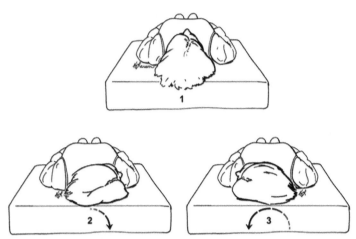

Fig. 5. Supine roll test. The patient's head is moved rapidly from the straight supine position (1) to the right side (2). Observe for horizontal nystagmus and note the direction and intensity. Then move the patient's head back to the straight position (1) for 15 seconds. Then move the head from straight to the head left position (3) and note any nystagmus and its direction and intensity. If the nystagmus is of the geotropic type, the side resulting in the strongest nystagmus is taken to be the affected side (see **Table 2**).

always beats horizontally, and may persist longer than the nystagmus of posterior canal BPPV. Consequently, patients may become nauseated with attempts to fatigue this form of BPPV. Identifying the affected side can be accomplished using the several methods listed in **Table 2** and proper lateralization is important to select correctly the appropriated treatment maneuver. In cases where the horizontal canal BPPV developed as the result of canal switch during treatment for posterior canal BPPV, then it is very probable to be the same ear as was affected by the posterior canal BPPV.

Treatment
There is no single, widely accepted method for treating horizontal canal BPPV. Indeed, there has been a proliferation of maneuvers to treat horizontal canal BPPV and many

Table 2		
Methods to aid in lateralizing horizontal canal benign paroxysmal positional vertigo (BPPV) to the affected side		
Provocative Maneuver	**Geotropic-Type Nystagmus (Presumed Canalolithiasis)**	**Apogeotropic-Type Nystagmus (Presumed Cupulolithiasis)**
Supine head roll test	Intensity of nystagmus strongest with head turned to affected side	Intensity of nystagmus stronger with head turned to unaffected side
Lie the patient straight back from the sitting to supine facing up	Horizontal nystagmus beating to the unaffected ear	Horizontal nystagmus beating to the affected ear
Bend the head forward in the upright position	Horizontal nystagmus beating to the affected ear	Horizontal nystagmus beating to the unaffected ear

Adapted from von Brevern M. Benign paroxysmal positional vertigo. Semin Neurol 2013;33:206; with permission.

studies trying to compare them. Several treatments seem to be reasonably effective for the horizontal canal BPPV. As a general principle, converting the horizontal canal BPPV from the apogeotropic to the geotropic form may make it more amenable to various treatment maneuvers.[45,46]

Lempert 360° roll maneuver Attempts to treat horizontal canal BPPV with the same maneuver used for posterior canal BPPV is likely to be unsuccessful.[47,48] The 360° roll or so-called Lempert maneuver[44–46,48] begins with the patient on his back, facing up. Sometimes, the affected side is unclear despite attempts to discern it using the methods given in **Table 2**. In these cases, 1 side can be picked at random and later the other side can be treated as well. With the head turned so that the affected ear is down or alternatively in the straight, face up supine position, the head is turned quickly 90° toward the unaffected side. A series of 90° turns toward the unaffected side is then undertaken sequentially until the patient has turned 360° and is back to the affected, ear-down position (**Fig. 6**). Once the final turns have been made, the patient is brought upright again. Each head position should be held for about 20 seconds, even when the nystagmus continues. Waiting longer does no harm, but may lead to the patient developing nausea and the shorter interval does not seem to diminish the likelihood of success.

Forced prolonged positioning Forced prolonged positioning, as the name implies, entails the patient lying down quickly from the sitting position to the unaffected side followed and then maintaining or "forcing" this position for 12 hours before the patient sits up again. Although there are no studies to indicate minimum amount of time

Lempert Roll Maneuver

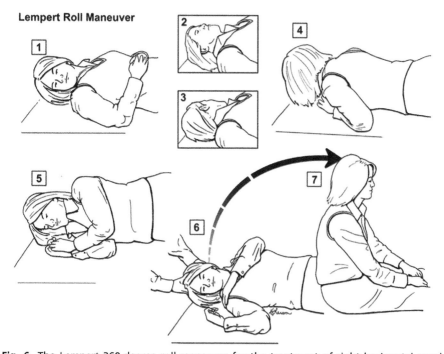

Fig. 6. The Lempert 360-degree roll maneuver for the treatment of right horizontal canal benign paroxysmal positional vertigo with geotropic-type nystagmus. The Lempert 360-degree roll maneuver for the treatment of right horizontal canal benign paroxysmal positional vertigo with geotropic-type nystagmus. Numbers 1–7 depict the sequential steps in the maneuver.

necessary to be successful, the original description was for 12 hours.[49] It seems likely that 5 to 10 minutes would achieve adequate sedimentation of the debris and is far more practical for patients than holding a position for 12 hours. This method may be something to consider for patients with more refractory horizontal canal BPPV.[45,50] Using forced prolonged positioning, remission rates range from 70% to 90%.[12,29,45,49]

Gufoni maneuver Variations of the Gufoni maneuver (**Fig. 7**) may be effective in treating both the geotropic and the apogeotropic forms of horizontal BPPV.[50,51] One study found that the Gufoni maneuver was successful in more than 80% of patients.[52] A class II, randomized, sham-controlled trial of 157 patients with apogeotropic horizontal canal BPPV found that the Gufoni maneuver was more effective (73%) than a sham maneuver that resulted in a 35% response rate (P<.001) at 1 hour and also at 1 month after treatment.[53] It is noteworthy that the response to sham was so high, suggesting that either the sham maneuver might have treated some patients or that horizontal canal BPPV has a propensity to resolve spontaneously.

Other maneuvers For treatment of the apogeotropic form of horizontal canal BPPV, there is a maneuver in which the head is shaken at 3 Hz (quite rapidly) for 15 seconds while the patient is supine with the head tilted forward about 30° that results in 37% to 47% response rates.[53,54] This maneuver may have some effectiveness by simply

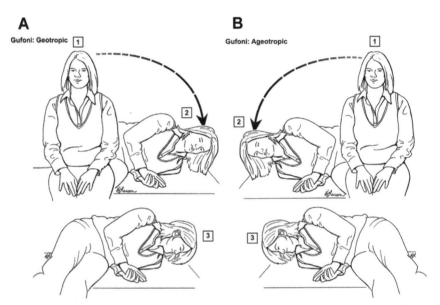

Fig. 7. The Gufoni maneuver illustrated is to treat right-sided horizontal canal benign paroxysmal positional vertigo (BPPV) that is geotropic (*A*) or apogeotropic (*B*). Numbers 1–3 depict the sequential steps in each maneuver. For the geotropic nystagmus type of lateral canal BPPV, the patient is taken from the sitting position to the straight side-lying position on the unaffected side (left in this case) and held in that position for 1 minute. The patient's head is quickly turned toward the ground about 60° and held in the position for 1 minute. The patient then sits up again with the head held toward the left shoulder until sitting upright again. For right horizontal canal BPPV with apogeotropic-type nystagmus, the patient is taken from the sitting position to the straight side-lying position on the unaffected side (right in this instance) for 1 minute. Then the patient's head is quickly turned 60° toward the ground and held in the position for 1 minute. The patient then sits up again, keeping the head held toward the right shoulder until fully upright.

promoting some otolith movements in the plane of the horizontal canals. There are other maneuvers and various permutations of them and some comparative studies. One thing they all have in common is a moderate rate of success and a moderate rate of improvement in the untreated group.

Authors' commentary The multitude of treatments described to treat horizontal canal BPPV is unnecessarily confusing. The 360° Lempert roll ("log roll" or "barbecue roll") seems as effective as any of the other methods. In fact, it may be that any kind of movement of the head hastens resolution of symptoms because the otolithic material is usually mechanically predisposed to moving out of the horizontal canal and back into the main vestibule. It may be sufficient to treat with the roll maneuver or the Gufoni maneuver and, if the symptoms persist in the course of daily activities by 48 hours, to advise the patient to sleep on the unaffected ear (forced prolonged positioning). Horizontal canal BPPV seems to self-resolve with greater frequency and more quickly[55] than does posterior canal BPPV, and even the latter often resolves in time. About 90% of cases of apogeotropic horizontal canal BPPV resolved in 1 study within 1 week and all had resolved by 4 weeks in several studies.[54,56]

Anterior Canal Benign Paroxysmal Positional Vertigo

Anterior canal BPPV is the least commonly encountered and in many cases is it seen only as a transient state from canal switch during the course of treating BPPV. The anterior canal is oriented in a position that makes otolithic material unlikely to enter the canal and even less likely to remain there. BPPV affecting the anterior canal is characterized by brief downbeating nystagmus with only a minor rotational component after Dix Hallpike positioning, no matter to which side the head is turned to (see **Table 1**).[23,25,44,56–58] Thus, the side of the diagnostic positioning maneuver is not helpful to reveal the side of the affected anterior canal. Theoretically, the affected side can be deduced from the torsional component of nystagmus, but this component can be fairly subtle in many cases, making it difficult to lateralize reliably without more sophisticated 3-dimensional eye movement recordings.[23,59–62]

Central positional downbeat nystagmus may be seen with lesions of the central vestibular pathways in the caudal cerebellum, so if there is doubt about the diagnosis, brain imaging with MRI should be undertaken particularly because this form of downbeating nystagmus usually self-resolves within a few days.[8,57]

Treatment

Anterior canal BPPV is rare and, as mentioned, usually resolves quickly so no established treatment maneuvers have been established by randomized trials. Anterior canal BPPV may be treated using any of the maneuvers that treat posterior BPPV,[63] although it may at times be unclear which side is affected. Another approach that avoids the need to identify the affected side is to position the patient from the sitting to the straight head hanging position with a modest degree of neck hyperextension and holding the position for 30 to 60 seconds. Then the head is flexed forward and the patient sits up.[12,60,64]

PROGNOSIS

Treatments for posterior canal BPPV are highly effective in the range of 90%[28,29,65] and a number needed to treat for BPPV using the canalith repositioning procedure is a remarkably low (1.4–1.6).[66] The number needed to treat is a statistical measurement of the number of patients who must be treated to achieve improvement in 1 patient. Improvement in this case is complete resolution of symptoms. Consequently this means that for every 3 patients with BPPV treated with canalith repositioning procedure, 2 have complete elimination of symptoms. This is one of the most highly effective treatments in all of clinical medicine. By comparison, the number needed to treat with pregabalin for even a 50% reduction in pain in fibromyalgia is 7.1 to 21.0.[67]

Recurrences of BPPV most commonly occur in the first year after onset and long-term recurrence rates range from 30% to 50% depending on the duration of follow-up.[65,68,69]

BENIGN PAROXYSMAL POSITIONAL VERTIGO IN THE EMERGENCY DEPARTMENT

Emergency department management of BPPV throughout most of the United States is still primarily focused on symptom management. A retrospective study of 20 patients previously revealed the lack of recognition of classical findings and lack of treatment making care cost inefficient.[70] It has now been 7 years since the publication of 2 separate practice guidelines establishing highly effective treatment maneuvers for the most common form of BPPV, but most patients seen in the emergency department continue to undergo head imaging studies and are given meclizine.[71] Patients with BPPV often present to the emergency department, but the diagnosis of Dix Hallpike maneuver to confirm the diagnosis is done in fewer than 4% of cases.[72] Indeed, the increasing cost of emergency department management of dizziness seems to stem from both an increase in the presentation of dizziness and to the increasing use of imaging studies.[73,74]

The last decade has shown that patients with vertebrobasilar stroke may present with isolated vertigo and the differentiation between a central and a peripheral cause of vertigo in the emergency department is of paramount importance. In a prospective study of 100 consecutive patients with positional nystagmus, the vast majority (80%) had BPPV and only 12% clearly had a central vestibular disorder.[75] An accurate clinical examination can almost always identify a central positional vertigo syndrome. As a rule, a central lesion should be suspected when any clinical feature of positional nystagmus differs from BPPV, including direction, duration, time course, and fatigability of nystagmus.[76] Central positional nystagmus is most often downbeating and (in contrast with anterior canal BPPV) typically lasts as long as the head is kept in the critical position. Fortunately, a central vestibular lesion imitating the characteristic pattern of posterior canal BPPV has not been reported convincingly to our knowledge. Some caution is required when horizontal positional nystagmus is observed, because patients with central lesions imitating BPPV of the horizontal canal have been described only rarely.[77,78] Most challenging is the differentiation of anterior canal BPPV presenting with transient downbeating positional nystagmus from a central cause and it is mandatory to exclude central nervous system disease by cerebral imaging if this nystagmus does not cease promptly after therapeutic maneuvers.

In 1 study of 26 patients, 15 were treated with canalith repositioning procedure and 11 with antivertiginous medications. Using the 2-hour endpoints of nausea and dizziness, there were no differences between the canalith repositioning group and the medication group.[79] One might question whether nausea and dizziness in patients sitting quietly on a gurney for several hours is the ideal endpoint for a condition that produces symptoms only with positional provocation. This is particularly true considering there were equally high patient satisfaction ratings, but 9 of the 26 sought additional care for the vertigo within 30 days.

SUMMARY

BPPV is a common cause of dizziness that presents to the emergency department owing to its sudden and often alarming onset. It is caused by movement of calcium carbonate material within the semicircular canals of the inner ear, triggering intense but fairly brief vertigo in response to head position changes, such as turning in bed or tilting one's head back. The Dix Hallpike maneuver should be undertaken in patients with a history of sudden brief spells of vertigo. The diagnosis can be confirmed by observing intense nystagmus in response to the positioning maneuver. Two highly effective treatment maneuvers can eliminate symptoms in about 90% of patients and, whenever possible, this treatment should be offered to patients, preferably by the clinician diagnosing the condition. Effective and timely treatment alleviates symptoms, improves patient productivity and quality of life, and is very cost efficient relative to deferring treatment to others in the outpatient setting or simply assuring the patient that symptoms are likely to subside eventually.

REFERENCES

1. Katsarkas A, Kirkham TH. Paroxysmal positional vertigo—a study of 255 cases. J Otolaryngol 1978;7:320–30.
2. Kollén L, Frändin K, Möller M, et al. Benign paroxysmal positional vertigo is a common cause of dizziness and unsteadiness in a large population of 75-year-olds. Aging Clin Exp Res 2012;24:317–23.
3. Oghalai JS, Manolidis S, Barth JL, et al. Unrecognized benign paroxysmal positional vertigo in elderly patients. Otolaryngol Head Neck Surg 2000;122:630–4.
4. von Brevern M, Radtke A, Lezius F, et al. Epidemiology of benign paroxysmal positional vertigo: a population based study. J Neurol Neurosurg Psychiatry 2007; 78:710–5.
5. Baloh RW, Honrubia V, Jacobson K. Benign positional vertigo: clinical and oculographic features in 240 cases. Neurology 1987;37:371–8.
6. Fife TD. Posttraumatic vertigo and dizziness. Semin Neurol 2013;33:238–43.
7. Motin M, Keren O, Groswasser Z, et al. Benign paroxysmal positional vertigo as the cause of dizziness in patients after severe traumatic brain injury: diagnosis and treatment. Brain Inj 2005;19:693–7.
8. Fife TD. Positional dizziness. Continuum (Minneap Minn) 2012;18(5 Neuro-otology): 1060–85.
9. Karlberg M, Halmagyi GM, Buttner U, et al. Sudden unilateral hearing loss with simultaneous ipsilateral posterior semicircular canal benign paroxysmal positional vertigo: a variant of vestibulo-cochlear neurolabyrinthitis? Arch Otolaryngol Head Neck Surg 2000;126:1024–9.
10. Brandt T, Steddin S. Current view of the mechanisms of benign paroxysmal positioning vertigo: cupulolithiasis or canalolithiasis? J Vestib Res 1993;3:373–82.
11. Baloh RW, Yue Q, Jacobson KM, et al. Persistent direction-changing positional nystagmus: another variant of benign positional vertigo? Neurology 1995;45: 1297–301.
12. von Brevern M. Benign paroxysmal positional vertigo. Semin Neurol 2013;33: 204–11.
13. Otsuka K, Negishi M, Suzuki M, et al. Experimental study on the aetiology of benign paroxysmal positional vertigo due to canalolithiasis: comparison between normal and vestibular dysfunction models. J Laryngol Otol 2014;128:68–72.
14. Nakahara H, Yoshimura E, Tsuda Y, et al. Damaged utricular function clarified by oVEMP in patients with benign paroxysmal positional vertigo. Acta Otolaryngol 2013;133:144–9.
15. Squires TM, Weidman MS, Hain TC, et al. A mathematical model for top-shelf vertigo: the role of sedimenting otoconia in BPPV. J Biomech 2004;37:1137–46.

16. Jang YS, Hwang CH, Shin JY, et al. Age-related changes on the morphology of the otoconia. Laryngoscope 2006;116:996–1001.
17. Walther LE, Wenzel A, Buder J, et al. Detection of human utricular otoconia degeneration in vital specimen and implications for benign paroxysmal positional vertigo. Eur Arch Otorhinolaryngol 2014;271:3133–8.
18. Yu S, Liu F, Cheng Z, et al. Association between osteoporosis and benign paroxysmal positional vertigo: a systematic review. BMC Neurol 2014;14:110–6.
19. Vibert D, Sans A, Kompis M, et al. Ultrastructural changes in otoconia of osteoporotic rats. Audiol Neurootol 2008;13:293–301.
20. Parham K, Leonard G, Feinn RS, et al. Prospective clinical investigation of the relationship between idiopathic benign paroxysmal positional vertigo and bone turnover: a pilot study. Laryngoscope 2013;123:2834–9.
21. Gizzi MS, Peddareddygari LR, Grewal RP. A familial form of benign paroxysmal positional vertigo maps to chromosome 15. Int J Neurosci 2014. [Epub ahead of print].
22. Lin GC, Basura GJ, Wong HT, et al. Canal switch after canalith repositioning procedure for benign paroxysmal positional vertigo. Laryngoscope 2012;122:2076–8.
23. Aw ST, Todd MJ, Aw GE, et al. Benign positional nystagmus. A study of its three-dimensional spatio-temporal characteristics. Neurology 2005;64:1897–905.
24. Nakayama M, Epley JM. BPPV and variants: improved treatment results with automated, nystagmus-based repositioning. Otolaryngol Head Neck Surg 2005;133:107–12.
25. Lopez-Escamez JA, Molina MI, Gamiz MJ, et al. Multiple positional nystagmus suggests multiple canal involvement in benign paroxysmal positional vertigo. Acta Otolaryngol 2005;125:954–61.
26. Fife TD. Benign paroxysmal positional vertigo. Semin Neurol 2009;29:500–8.
27. Katsarkas A. Benign paroxysmal positional vertigo (BPPV): idiopathic versus post-traumatic. Acta Otolaryngol 1999;119:745–9.
28. Fife TD, Iverson DJ, Lempert T, et al. Quality Standards Subcommittee, American Academy of Neurology. Practice parameter: therapies for benign paroxysmal positional vertigo (an evidence-based review): report of the Quality Standards Subcommittee of the American Academy of Neurology. Neurology 2008;70:2067–74.
29. Bhattacharyya N, Baugh RF, Orvidas L, et al. Clinical practice guideline: benign paroxysmal positional vertigo. Otolaryngol Head Neck Surg 2008;139(5 Suppl 4): S47–81.
30. Mandalà M, Santoro GP, Asprella Libonati G, et al. Double-blind randomized trial on short-term efficacy of the Semont maneuver for the treatment of posterior canal benign paroxysmal positional vertigo. J Neurol 2012;259:882–5.
31. Chen Y, Zhuang J, Zhang L, et al. Short-term efficacy of Semont maneuver for benign paroxysmal positional vertigo: a double-blind randomized trial. Otol Neurotol 2012;33:1127–30.
32. Semont A, Freyss G, Vitte E. Curing the BPPV with a liberatory maneuver. Adv Otorhinolaryngol 1988;42:290–3.
33. Tirelli G, D'Orlando E, Giacomarra V, et al. Benign positional vertigo without detectable nystagmus. Laryngoscope 2001;111:1053–6.
34. Haynes DS, Resser JR, Labadie RF, et al. Treatment of benign positional vertigo using the Semont maneuver: efficacy in patients presenting without nystagmus. Laryngoscope 2002;112:796–801.
35. Horii A, Kitahara T, Osaki Y, et al. Intractable benign paroxysmal positioning vertigo: long-term follow-up and inner ear abnormality detected by three-dimensional magnetic resonance imaging. Otol Neurotol 2010;31(2):250–5.

36. Teggi R, Giordano L, Bondi S, et al. Residual dizziness after successful repositioning maneuvers for idiopathic benign paroxysmal positional vertigo in the elderly. Eur Arch Otorhinolaryngol 2011;268:507–11.
37. Pollak L, Segal P, Stryier R, et al. Beliefs and emotional reactions in patients with benign paroxysmal positional vertigo: a longitudinal study. Am J Otolaryngol 2012;33:221–5.
38. Hunt WT, Zimmermann EF, Hilton MP. Modifications of the Epley (canalith repositioning) manoeuvre for posterior canal benign paroxysmal positional vertigo (BPPV). Cochrane Database Syst Rev 2012;(4):CD008675.
39. Tanimoto H, Doi K, Katata K, et al. Self-treatment for benign paroxysmal positional vertigo of the posterior semicircular canal. Neurology 2005;65:1299–300.
40. Radtke A, von Brevern M, Tiel-Wilck K, et al. Self-treatment of benign paroxysmal positional vertigo: Semont maneuver vs Epley procedure. Neurology 2004;63: 150–2.
41. Kerber KA, Burke JF, Skolarus LE, et al. A prescription for the Epley maneuver: www.youtube.com? Neurology 2012;79:376–80.
42. Kerber KA, Skolarus LE, Callaghan BC, et al. Consumer demand for online dizziness information: if you build it, they may come. Front Neurol 2014;5:50.
43. Pagnini P, Nuti D, Vannucchi P. Benign paroxysmal vertigo of the horizontal canal. ORL J Otorhinolaryngol Relat Spec 1989;51:161–70.
44. Fife T. Recognition and management of horizontal canal benign positional vertigo. Am J Otol 1998;19:345–51.
45. Casani AP, Vannucci G, Fattori B, et al. The treatment of horizontal canal positional vertigo: our experience in 66 cases. Laryngoscope 2002;112:172–8.
46. Baloh RW, Jacobson BA, Honrubia V. Horizontal semicircular canal variant of benign positional vertigo. Neurology 1993;43:2542–9.
47. Herdman SJ, Tusa RJ. Complications of the canalith repositioning procedure. Arch Otolaryngol Head Neck Surg 1996;122:281–6.
48. Lempert T, Tiel-Wilck K. A positional maneuver for treatment of horizontal-canal benign positional vertigo. Laryngoscope 1998;106:476–8.
49. Vannucchi P, Giannoni B, Pagnini P. Treatment of horizontal semicircular canal benign paroxysmal positional vertigo. J Vestib Res 1997;7:1–6.
50. Gufoni M, Mastrosimone L, Di Nasso F. Trattamento con manovra di riposizionatmento per la canalolitiasi orizzontale. Acta Otorhinolaryngol Ital 1998;18: 363–7.
51. Mandalà M, Pepponi E, Santoro GP, et al. Double-blind randomized trial on the efficacy of the Gufoni maneuver for treatment of lateral canal BPPV. Laryngoscope 2013;123:1782–6.
52. Riggio F, Dispenza F, Gallina S, et al. Management of benign paroxysmal positional vertigo of lateral semicircular canal by Gufoni's manoeuvre. Am J Otolaryngol 2009;30:106–11.
53. Kim JS, Oh SY, Lee SH, et al. Randomized clinical trial for apogeotropic horizontal canal benign paroxysmal positional vertigo. Neurology 2012;78:159–66.
54. Oh SY, Kim JS, Jeong SH, et al. Treatment of apogeotropic benign positional vertigo: comparison of therapeutic head-shaking and modified Semont maneuver. J Neurol 2009;256:1330–6.
55. Lee SH, Kim JS. Benign paroxysmal positional vertigo. J Clin Neurol 2010;6: 51–63.
56. Imai T, Takeda N, Ito M, et al. Natural course of positional vertigo in patients with apogeotropic variant of horizontal canal benign paroxysmal positional vertigo. Auris Nasus Larynx 2011;38:2–5.

57. Bertholon P, Bronstein AM, Davies RA, et al. Positional down beating nystagmus in 50 patients: cerebellar disorders and possible anterior semicircular canalithiasis. J Neurol Neurosurg Psychiatry 2002;72:366–72.

58. Brantberg K, Bergenius J. Treatment of anterior benign paroxysmal positional vertigo by canal plugging: a case report. Acta Otolaryngol 2002;122:28–30.

59. Cambi J, Astore S, Mandalà M, et al. Natural course of positional down-beating nystagmus of peripheral origin. J Neurol 2013;260:1489–96.

60. Casani AP, Cerchiai N, Dallan I, et al. Anterior canal lithiasis: diagnosis and treatment. Otolaryngol Head Neck Surg 2011;144:412–8.

61. Imai T, Takeda N, Ito M, et al. 3D analysis of benign positional nystagmus due to cupulolithiasis in posterior semicircular canal. Acta Otolaryngol 2009;129:1044–9.

62. Korres S, Riga M, Balatsouras D, et al. Benign paroxysmal positional vertigo of the anterior canal: atypical clinical findings and possible underlying mechanisms. Int J Audiol 2008;47:276–82.

63. Kim YK, Shin JE, Chung JW. The effect of canalolith repositioning for anterior semicircular canal canalolithiasis. ORL J Otorhinolaryngol Relat Spec 2005;67: 56–60.

64. Yacovino DA, Hain TC, Gualtieri F. New therapeutic maneuver for anterior canal benign paroxysmal positional vertigo. J Neurol 2009;256:1851–5.

65. Nunez RA, Cass SP, Furman JM. Short- and long-term outcomes of canalith repositioning for benign paroxysmal positional vertigo. Otolaryngol Head Neck Surg 2000;122:647–52.

66. Brown MD. Is the canalith repositioning maneuver effective in the acute management of benign positional vertigo? Ann Emerg Med 2011;58:286–7.

67. Moore RA, Straube S, Wiffen PJ, et al. Pregabalin for acute and chronic pain in adults. Cochrane Database Syst Rev 2009;(3):CD007076.

68. Hain TC, Helminski JO, Reis IL, et al. Vibration does not improve results of the canalith repositioning procedure. Arch Otolaryngol Head Neck Surg 2000;126: 617–22.

69. Sakaida M, Takeuchi K, Ishinaga H, et al. Long-term outcome of benign paroxysmal positional vertigo. Neurology 2003;60:1532–4.

70. Fife D, Fitzgerald JE. Do patients with benign paroxysmal positional vertigo receive prompt treatment? Analysis of waiting times and human and financial costs associated with current practice. Int J Audiol 2005;44:50–7.

71. Newman-Toker DE, Camargo CA Jr, Hsieh YH, et al. Disconnect between charted vestibular diagnoses and emergency department management decisions: a cross-sectional analysis from a nationally representative sample. Acad Emerg Med 2009;16:970–7.

72. Kerber KA, Burke JF, Skolarus LE, et al. Use of BPPV processes in emergency department dizziness presentations: a population-based study. Otolaryngol Head Neck Surg 2013;148:425–30.

73. Saber Tehrani AS, Coughlan D, Hsieh YH, et al. Rising annual costs of dizziness presentations to U.S. emergency departments. Acad Emerg Med 2013;20: 689–96.

74. Ahsan SF, Syamal MN, Yaremchuk K, et al. The costs and utility of imaging in evaluating dizzy patients in the emergency room. Laryngoscope 2013;123: 2250–3.

75. Bertholon P, Tringali S, Fay MB, et al. Prospective study of positional nystagmus in 100 consecutive patients. Ann Otol Rhinol Laryngol 2006;115:587–94.

76. Büttner U, Helmchen C, Brandt T. Diagnostic criteria for central versus peripheral positioning nystagmus and vertigo: a review. Acta Otolaryngol 1999;119(1):1–5.

77. Bassani R, Della Torre S. Positional nystagmus reversing from geotropic to apogetropic: a new central vestibular syndrome. J Neurol 2011;258:313–5.
78. Kim JS, Oh SY, Lee SH, et al. Randomized clinical trial for geotropic horizontal canal benign paroxysmal positional vertigo. Neurology 2012;79:700–7.
79. Sacco RR, Burmeister DB, Rupp VA. Management of benign paroxysmal positional vertigo: a randomized controlled trial. J Emerg Med 2014;46:575–81.

Early Diagnosis and Management of Acute Vertigo from Vestibular Migraine and Ménière's Disease

 CrossMark

Barry Seemungal, BSc, MB BCh, PhD, FRCP[a],*, Diego Kaski, MBBS, PhD[a],
Jose Antonio Lopez-Escamez, MD, PhD[b]

KEYWORDS

- Vestibular disorders • Vertigo • Hearing loss • Tinnitus • Migraine
- Ménière's disease

KEY POINTS

- Vestibular migraine (VM) is second only to benign paroxysmal positional vertigo as the most common cause of acute episodic vestibular symptoms.
- Ménière's disease (MD) is uncommon; however, accurate diagnosis (or its exclusion) enables the correct management of patients with acute episodic vestibular symptoms.
- A focused neurologic examination can exclude other sinister causes such as stroke.
- Although most cases can be treated in the emergency room (ER), some patients may require a brief hospital admission to control symptoms.

VESTIBULAR MIGRAINE
Case Scenario

A 46-year old woman presented with a 2-hour history of sudden onset and continuous vertigo (a feeling that her head was spinning) and severe nausea but mild occipital headache. During the previous 4 months, she noted weekly uncomfortable headaches occasionally accompanied by photophobia, bilateral tinnitus, and aural fullness. In her late teens to mid-20s, she suffered from monthly severe headaches with nausea, vomiting, and sometimes severe dizziness, lasting up to 2 days. On this occasion, the clinical examination was entirely normal, including a normal gait. MRI of the brain showed normal findings. She was treated with intravenous prochlorperazine and oral aspirin and discharged with a prescription of oral propranolol 20 mg twice a day with a plan for a clinic follow-up in 8 weeks.

[a] Division of Brain Sciences, Charing Cross Hospital, Imperial College London, London, W6 8RF, UK; [b] Otology and Neurotology Group CTS495, Department of Otolaryngology, Hospital de Poniente, El Ejido, Almería, Spain
* Corresponding author.
E-mail address: b.seemungal@imperial.ac.uk

Neurol Clin 33 (2015) 619–628
http://dx.doi.org/10.1016/j.ncl.2015.04.008
0733-8619/15/$ – see front matter © 2015 Elsevier Inc. All rights reserved.
neurologic.theclinics.com

Prevalence and Pathophysiologic Mechanisms

VM has an estimated lifetime prevalence of approximately 3.2%, making it one of the most common vestibular disorders.[1] The estimated 1-year prevalence is 0.89% across the population[2] and 5% in women aged 40 to 54 years.[3]

The current understanding and hypotheses underlying the pathophysiology of VM stem from genetic and in vitro studies, animal models, and human clinical studies of migraine.[4–8] A key mechanism identified in migraine pathophysiology is activation of the trigeminovascular system. The labyrinthine vessels are innervated by trigeminal nerve terminals, which, combined with the presence of vasoactive neuropeptides in the perivascular afferent terminals of these trigeminal fibers, support the notion that the vascular, neuroinflammatory, and central neural mechanisms implicated in migraine are common to the central vestibular mechanisms and to the inner ear.[9,10] This notion may explain why there exists a reciprocal interaction between peripheral vestibular deficits and VM.[11,12]

Neuroanatomic regions implicated

Numerous brain regions and networks have been implicated in the pathogenesis of VM, including the posterior and anterior insula, orbitofrontal cortex, and the posterior and anterior cingulate gyri.[13–15] The perceptual correlate of VM encompasses vestibular thalamocortical networks that produce perceptual responses to vestibular, visual, proprioceptive, and somatosensory afferent inputs. This cognitive-behavioral domain includes frontal and parietal cortical pathways related to premonitory symptoms associated with balance control.[16]

Brainstem pathways have been implicated in the generation of somatic (eg, vestibular ocular and vestibular spinal reflexes) and visceral (vestibular sympathetic and parasympathetic) motor responses.[17] In the context of spontaneous migraine attacks, these vestibular sensorimotor responses seem to be modulated by the cerebellum.[18] Functional neuroimaging techniques suggest that VM relates to abnormal brain sensitization leading to a dysmodulation of multimodal sensory integration and processing resulting in a vestibulothalamocortical dysfunction.[19]

At the cellular level, it has been identified in animal models of migraine that activation of trigeminal ganglion innervation within cerebral and meningeal vasculature induces a trigeminovascular reflex-mediated vasodilation of meningeal vessels via the sphenopalatine ganglion.[20] Similar events have been observed in the murine inner ear.[21] The prevalence of VM suggests that multiple functional variants may confer a genetic susceptibility leading to a dysregulation of excitatory-inhibitory balance in brain structures involved in the processing of sensory information, vestibular inputs, and pain.[19]

At present, there is no convincing evidence to explain how migraine could cause an apparent episodic inner ear or central vestibular dysfunction as observed during acute VM.[22] Transient vasospasm of the blood supply to the inner ear (via the internal auditory artery) is one proposed hypothesis. Conversely, a transient episode of inner ear ischemia (from cerebrovascular disease) could trigger a migraine, a tenable possibility given the intimate link between the vestibular apparatus and the trigeminovascular system. Another explanation is the neurogenic hypothesis, for example, via a channelopathy that can manifest with migraines,[23] and such syndromes are associated with episodic neurologic dysfunction. A channelopathy hypothesis, as a common underlying mechanism, could explain the epidemiologic link between migraine and MD, perhaps also explaining the symptomatic overlap between MD and VM.[24]

Definitions and Diagnostic Criteria (Differentiation from transient ischaemic attack [TIA] + Approach to Initial Diagnosis)

The diagnosis of VM requires clinical suspicion. Recently, a consensus paper was published on the criteria for VM (**Box 1**).[27] The consensus acknowledges that migraine may present with mainly vestibular symptoms and hence is called VM. The criteria recognize the bidirectional relationship between migraine and vertigo (see note h in **Box 1**), that is, acute vertigo of any origin can trigger migraine features, including headache. Hence, patients with a primary vestibular problem who are also migraineurs, could at first glance conform to the VM criteria.

An important differential diagnosis of acute VM is of a cerebellar stroke not involving the brainstem. Although VM may present in a myriad of ways, with examination signs mimicking an acute or central peripheral vestibular syndrome,[22] the only real differential diagnosis of cerebellar stroke not involving the brainstem is an acute VM. Such strokes are typically embolic[28] and present with thunderclap onset vertigo (often severe) with nausea, vomiting, and imbalance on walking, and half the cases have occipital headache. The examination in such cerebellar strokes may show a direction-changing nystagmus on gaze testing and/or a skew deviation (see article elsewhere in this issue), both features of a central lesion. Some cases of cerebellar stroke not involving the brainstem may present with little or no eye signs.[29] The head impulse test is normal in 90% of cerebellar strokes.[30] Irrespective of the head impulse test, gait ataxia is a red flag directing the clinician to perform emergency neuroimaging.

In a patient presenting with vertigo for the first time, it may not be possible to clinically differentiate between acute VM and an acute cerebellar stroke because both may present with severe vertigo, nausea, vomiting, posterior headache, gait ataxia, few ocular signs, and a preserved head impulse test. In such cases, immediate brain MRI should be performed and possibly repeated if the initial scan is normal and the clinical suspicion is high. A history of multiple similar episodes over a prolonged period is likely to represent VM and not stroke however, on first presentation, such patients should be investigated with neuroimaging if the clinical picture warrants it.

In conclusion, although a cerebellar stroke not involving the brainstem may present in a manner identical to VM, it can be reliably distinguished from an acute peripheral vestibular syndrome (see article elsewhere in this issue). Hence, it perhaps is most important to consider the red flags for investigating such cases. VM can present with signs of a peripheral vestibular lesion; however, the need for immediate investigation is less pressing. The diagnosis of VM can be definitively made in cases presenting with repeated episodes (that conform to the VM diagnostic criteria) whereby no other vestibular diagnosis is forthcoming and in whom there are no interictal abnormalities. In contrast, patients with MD typically display persistent sensorineural hearing loss and impaired peripheral vestibular function in the affected ear even between attacks.

Bedside and Laboratory Diagnostic Tests

History

In acute VM, there may be no headache complaint; however, if present, it is important to characterize the type of headache during the attack. In addition, the clinician should ask about previous headache history. The headache interview should include specific questions concerning location (unilateral in migraine), pulsating quality, moderate or severe intensity, aggravation by activity, and sensitivity to light and sound. Although visual symptoms may occur, one would not expect any sensory deficit,

Box 1
Vestibular migraine diagnostic criteria

1. Definite vestibular migraine

   a. At least 5 episodes with vestibular symptoms[a] of moderate or severe intensity,[b] lasting 5 minutes to 72 hours[c]

   b. Current or previous history of migraine with or without aura according to the International Classification of Headache Disorders (ICHD)[d]

   c. One or more migraine features with at least 50% of the vestibular episodes[e]:

      i Headache with at least 2 of the following: (1) one-sided location, (2) pulsating quality, (3) moderate or severe pain intensity, (4) aggravation by routine physical activity

      ii Photophobia and phonophobia[f]

      iii Visual aura[g]

   d. Not better accounted for by another vestibular or ICHD diagnosis[h]

2. Probable vestibular migraine

   a. At least 5 episodes with vestibular symptoms[a] of moderate or severe intensity,[b] lasting 5 minutes to 72 hours[c]

   b. Only one of the criteria b and c for vestibular migraine is fulfilled (migraine history or migraine features during the episode)

   c. Not better accounted for by another vestibular or ICHD diagnosis[h]

[a] Vestibular symptoms, as defined by the Barany Society's Classification of Vestibular Symptoms[25] and qualifying for a diagnosis of vestibular migraine, include (1) spontaneous vertigo including internal vertigo, a false sensation of self-motion, and external vertigo, a false sensation that the visual surround is spinning or flowing; (2) positional vertigo, occurring after a change of head position; (3) visually induced vertigo, triggered by a complex or large moving visual stimulus; (4) head motion-induced vertigo, occurring during head motion; and (5) head motion-induced dizziness with nausea. Dizziness is characterized by a sensation of disturbed spatial orientation. Other forms of dizziness are currently not included in the classification of vestibular migraine.

[b] Vestibular symptoms are rated "moderate" when they interfere with but do not prohibit daily activities and "severe" if daily activities cannot be continued.

[c] Duration of episodes is highly variable: About 30% of patients have episodes lasting minutes, 30% have attacks for hours, and another 30% have attacks for several days. The remaining 10% have attacks lasting seconds only, which tend to occur repeatedly during head motion, visual stimulation, or after changes of head position. In these patients, episode duration is defined as the total period during which short attacks recur. At the other end of the spectrum, there are patients who may take 4 weeks to fully recover from an episode. However, the core episode rarely exceeds 72 hours.

[d] Migraine categories 1.1 and 1.2 of the ICDH.[26]

[e] One symptom is sufficient during a single episode. Different symptoms may occur during different episodes. Associated symptoms may occur before, during, or after the vestibular symptoms.

[f] Phonophobia is defined as sound-induced discomfort. It is a transient and bilateral phenomenon that must be differentiated from recruitment, which is often unilateral and persistent. Recruitment leads to an enhanced perception and often distortion of loud sounds in an ear with decreased hearing.

[g] Visual auras are characterized by bright scintillating lights or zigzag lines, often with a scotoma that interferes with reading. Visual auras typically expand from 5 to 20 minutes and last for less than 60 minutes. They are often, but not always, restricted to 1 hemifield. Other types of migraine aura, for example, somatosensory or dysphasic aura, are not included as diagnostic criteria because their phenomenology is less specific and most patients also have visual auras.

[h] History and physical examinations do not suggest another vestibular disorder, such a disorder is considered but ruled out by appropriate investigations, or such disorder is present as a comorbid or independent condition, but episodes can be clearly differentiated. Migraine attacks may be induced by vestibular stimulation.[11] Therefore, the differential diagnosis should include other vestibular disorders complicated by superimposed migraine attacks.

speech/language symptoms, or motor weakness in VM, although virtually any combination of transient neurologic features is possible as part of an acute migraine syndrome. Although hemorrhagic stroke is widely known to be associated with headache, it is less well recognized that occipital headache is a feature in one-third of acute posterior circulation ischemic stroke.[31] Hence, the presence of acute headache does not immediately include a diagnosis of VM to the exclusion of stroke.

The examination

The examination (see article elsewhere in this issue) should include an assessment of cranial nerves, eye movements including the cover test, vergence, spontaneous and gaze-evoked nystagmus assessment, saccades, smooth pursuit, and the head impulse test. When the neurologic examination indicates central dysfunction, then immediate neuroimaging is indicated looking for brainstem or cerebellar pathology. If brain MRI shows normal findings and the clinical suspicion is high, then the patient should be clinically monitored and reimaged because early MRI can miss acute brainstem infarction.

Laboratory test

Blood glucose levels are determined.

Immediate Treatment Options

There are no robust clinical trial data for the immediate treatment of VM; however, treatment is primarily symptomatic and hence follows standard medical practice such as fluid replacement for vomiting (eg, intravenous saline) and antiemetics for nausea (prochlorperazine, metoclopramide, or cyclizine). It is advisable to avoid excessive sedation, which precludes reliable monitoring of the neurologic state. In patients in whom hemorrhagic cerebellar stroke has been excluded, a single enteral dose of aspirin, 900 to 1200 mg, or nonsteroidal anti-inflammatory drug (eg, ibuprofen 400–800 mg) can be given for headache.

Triage and Disposition

Prophylaxis

In some patients, migraine triggers can be identified, such as lack of sleep or food, psychological stress, or certain foodstuffs (eg, chocolate or cheese). Lifestyle adjustments can reduce attack frequency by avoiding such triggers. In some patients, there are no obvious triggers, and when attacks are frequent, standard practice includes the use of a daily dose of an antimigraine drug to reduce the frequency of attacks. The evidence supporting the use of these drugs in VM is limited, but commonly used drugs include β-blockers (propanolol), tricyclic antidepressants (amitriptyline), antiepileptics (valproate, topiramate), and antiserotonergics (pizotifen).

Patients with poorly controlled VM often develop chronic maladaptive symptoms such as visually induced dizziness. The authors' practice is to first treat these patients with antimigraine prophylactic drugs and then add vestibular rehabilitation exercises after if not fully recovered.

MÉNIÈRE'S DISEASE

Case Scenario

A 39-year-old man presented to the ER with severe vertigo with nausea and vomiting. Four hours previously he had woken to find that there was a fullness in his right ear. An hour later, there was a ringing noise in his right ear followed by a distortion of hearing on the right. He had a gradual build-up of feeling that he was spinning around. Eventually, he began to see the room spin around and started to vomit. He came to the ER.

The patient reported that he had 2 similar attacks during the past year. On this occasion, the examination showed a left beating third-degree vestibular nystagmus but with a normal head impulse test. Twenty minutes later, the patient was reexamined, but now the nystagmus was beating to the patient's right. The patient was treated with parenteral prochlorperazine. His vertigo and nausea settled after 30 minutes. The patient was observed for a further 4 hours and then eventually allowed to go home with a 2-day supply of prochlorperazine.

Prevalence and Pathophysiologic Mechanisms

The prevalence of MD is 5 to 500 per 100,000 habitants, and familial MD is around 9% of cases.[32] Human temporal bone studies have linked MD symptoms to the accumulation of endolymph within the cochlear duct (scala media) and the sacculus in the inner ear. It is thought that this endolymphatic hydrops begins with derangement of the ionic composition of the scala media. However, current data support the hypothesis that endolymphatic hydrops is an epiphenomenon associated with a variety of inner ear disorders,[33] and familial clustering indicates that genetics and environmental factors contribute to its development.[32]

Definitions and Diagnostic Criteria (Differentiation from TIA + Approach to Initial Diagnosis)

MD is characterized by recurrent attacks of spontaneous vertigo associated with hearing loss and tinnitus in the same ear.[34] Aural fullness and headache can be found during the attacks. The International Classification for Vestibular Disorders Committee of the Barany Society has developed consensus diagnostic criteria with American Academy of Otolaryngology – Head and Neck Surgery, European Academy of Otology & Neuro-Otology, Japan Society for Equilibrium Research, and the Korean Balance Society.[35] These criteria define 2 categories: definite and probable MD (**Box 2**).

Bedside and Laboratory Diagnostic Tests

A national survey in the United States showed that only 26.9% to 46.7% of otolaryngologists relied on history, physical examination, and audiometry alone to diagnose MD. Adjunctive tests are thus helpful to support the clinical diagnosis, particularly given the high rates of misdiagnosis (mainly overdiagnosis) of MD.

A focused eye movement examination should evaluate the presence of spontaneous and gaze-evoked nystagmus, the integrity of the vestibular ocular reflex

---

Box 2
Ménière's disease diagnostic criteria

Definite Ménière's disease

1. Two or more spontaneous episodes of vertigo, each lasting 20 minutes to 12 hours
2. Audiometrically documented low- to medium-frequency sensorineural hearing loss in the affected ear on at least 1 occasion before, during, or after one of the episodes of vertigo
3. Fluctuating aural symptoms (hearing, tinnitus, or fullness) in the affected ear
4. Not better accounted for by another vestibular diagnosis

Probable Ménière's disease

1. Two or more episodes of vertigo or dizziness, each lasting 20 minutes to 24 hours
2. Fluctuating aural symptoms (hearing, tinnitus, or fullness) in the reported ear
3. Not better accounted for by another vestibular diagnosis

(head impulse test), pursuit, and saccadic eye movements. Positional maneuvers should be performed in any patient presenting with episodic dizziness to exclude benign paroxysmal positional vertigo.

A bedside assessment of hearing may be insufficient to identify hearing loss, and an audiogram should be obtained in any patient with suspected MD, including tympanometry. Hearing loss is usually in the low-frequency range, and MD can result in marked intolerance to loud sounds.[36] Hearing and tinnitus fluctuate in the early stages of disease, but in the later stages they may become permanent.

Brain imaging, ideally with MRI, helps one to exclude secondary causes of Ménière's syndrome and posterior fossa lesions that may present with progressive hearing loss and vertigo. Moreover, endolymphatic hydrops in Ménière's disease may be visualized on high-resolution MRI after transtympanic gadolinium injection.[37]

During electrocochleography (EChG), an evoked summating potential (SP) and action potential (AP) are recorded in response to click or tone burst stimuli recorded by an intratympanic or extratympanic electrode. In a large case series, increased SP/AP ratio (>0.4) was found in 72% of patients with a clinical diagnosis of MD,[38] and the yield of the test increases with disease severity and duration. Although not widely available in routine clinical practice, EChG can be of use, particularly when there exists diagnostic uncertainty.[39]

The cervical vestibular evoked myogenic potential (cVEMP) is a short latency inhibitory potential of the ipsilateral sternocleidomastoid muscle evoked by a brief and loud (>85 dB) monaural click or tone burst stimuli.[40] The cVEMP is thought to be of saccular origin and mediated by the inferior vestibular nerve.[40] Patients with MD have increased cVEMP thresholds or absent VEMPs compared with controls.[41] Consistent with its otolithic basis, abnormal cVEMPS are more common in patients with Tumarkin crises[42] and also seen in 27% of the contralateral asymptomatic ears of patients with MD.[43]

The role of oculography in the diagnosis of MD is limited but may help differentiate MD from central causes of vertigo. Although pathologic canal paresis is present in 42% to 73% of patients with MD,[44] complete loss of function is rare, and therefore, only a minority of patients have an impaired head impulse test.[44] Caloric testing may help in the assessment of contralateral function before an ablative procedure, evaluation of postablative residual function, and identification of patients with preserved ipsilesional canal function where nondestructive treatment options may be preferred.[45]

Immediate Treatment Options (Including Manipulative and Pharmacologic [Rehabilitative])

In an acute attack of MD, the treatment is symptomatic. Nausea and vomiting can be treated with standard antiemetics such as phenothiazines (prochlorperazine), antihistamines (cyclizine), and antimuscarinic drugs (scopolamine). It is reasonable to provide a benzodiazepine during the acute attack to alleviate anxiety.

Triage and Disposition

The natural history of Ménière's disease is unpredictable, although typically unilateral at onset, whereby the frequency of attacks first increases, then decreases. Bilateral involvement is more common with increasing disease duration: 15% in the first 2 years, 35% after 10 years, and up to 47% after 20 years.[46]

Various interventions are used to reduce the number of attacks or progression of audiovestibular failure in MD, although none have a strong evidence base.[34] One intervention is dietary salt restriction (daily sodium intake of <2 g/d), which is thought to reduce the osmotic build-up of pressure in the endolymphatic compartment. Using a similar logic, diuretics are also prescribed for MD, although a Cochrane review did not support their use.[47] High-dose betahistine may have a prophylactic effect on the frequency of attacks of MD, at least in the first year,[48] although its effect on vestibular and audiological function is unknown. Although the evidence remains scarce, systemic steroids should be considered in patients with a comorbid autoimmune condition especially if there is bilateral sensorineural hearing loss.[49] There is also weak evidence that intratympanic dexamethasone may reduce attacks of Ménière's disease and without significant systemic side effects.[50,51] In patients in whom there is significant audiovestibular loss in the affected ear but with continuing severe attacks, subablative therapy with intratympanic gentamicin may be effective in curtailing attacks.[34] Finally, the role of vestibular rehabilitation in the acute phase of the disease is controversial, given the fluctuating nature of vestibular symptoms in these patients. Nevertheless, there is evidence to suggest that vestibular rehabilitation across the spectrum of MD improves both subjective and objective balance function.[52]

When to refer

Specialist referral is indicated in patients with clinically suspected MD for diagnostic purposes. Such patients may also require referral for consideration of preventative strategies, for medical and surgical intervention where symptoms are persistent or severe, and to ensure the involvement of a multidisciplinary team, including otolaryngologists, neuro-otologists, physiotherapists, and audiologists. Given the unpredictable and disabling nature of the condition, psychological support can play an important role in long-term management to improve quality of life.

REFERENCES

1. Lempert T, Neuhauser H. Epidemiology of vertigo, migraine and vestibular migraine. J Neurol 2009;256(3):333–8.
2. Neuhauser HK, Radtke A, von Brevern M, et al. Migrainous vertigo: prevalence and impact on quality of life. Neurology 2006;67(6):1028–33.
3. Hsu LC, Wang SJ, Fuh JL. Prevalence and impact of migrainous vertigo in midlife women: a community-based study. Cephalalgia 2011;31(1):77–83.
4. Goadsby PJ, Lipton RB, Ferrari MD. Migraine – current understanding and treatment. N Engl J Med 2002;346(4):257–70.
5. Pietrobon D. Migraine: new molecular mechanisms. Neuroscientist 2005;11(4): 373–86.
6. Pietrobon D, Moskowitz MA. Pathophysiology of migraine. Annu Rev Physiol 2013;75:365–91.
7. Vecchia D, Pietrobon D. Migraine: a disorder of brain excitatory-inhibitory balance? Trends Neurosci 2012;35(8):507–20.
8. von Brevern M, Radtke A, Clarke AH, et al. Migrainous vertigo presenting as episodic positional vertigo. Neurology 2004;62(3):469–72.
9. May A, Goadsby PJ. The trigeminovascular system in humans: pathophysiologic implications for primary headache syndromes of the neural influences on the cerebral circulation. J Cereb Blood Flow Metab 1999;19(2):115–27.
10. Vass Z, Dai CF, Steyger PS, et al. Co-localization of the vanilloid capsaicin receptor and substance P in sensory nerve fibers innervating cochlear and vertebro-basilar arteries. Neuroscience 2004;124(4):919–27.
11. Murdin L, Davies RA, Bronstein AM. Vertigo as a migraine trigger. Neurology 2009;73(8):638–42.
12. Seemungal B, Rudge P, Davies R, et al. Three patients with migraine following caloric-induced vestibular stimulation. J Neurol 2006;253(8):1000–1.

13. Bucher SF, Dieterich M, Wiesmann M, et al. Cerebral functional magnetic resonance imaging of vestibular, auditory, and nociceptive areas during galvanic stimulation. Ann Neurol 1998;44(1):120–5.

14. Dieterich M, Brandt T. Functional brain imaging of peripheral and central vestibular disorders. Brain 2008;131(Pt 10):2538–52.

15. Fasold O, von Brevern M, Kuhberg M, et al. Human vestibular cortex as identified with caloric stimulation in functional magnetic resonance imaging. Neuroimage 2002;17(3):1384–93.

16. Furman JM, Marcus DA, Balaban CD. Vestibular migraine: clinical aspects and pathophysiology. Lancet Neurol 2013;12(7):706–15.

17. Holstein GR, Friedrich VL Jr, Kang T, et al. Direct projections from the caudal vestibular nuclei to the ventrolateral medulla in the rat. Neuroscience 2011;175:104–17.

18. Afridi SK, Giffin NJ, Kaube H, et al. A positron emission tomographic study in spontaneous migraine. Arch Neurol 2005;62(8):1270–5.

19. Espinosa-Sánchez JM, Lopez-Escamez JA. New insights into pathophysiology of vestibular migraine. Front Neurol 2015;6:12.

20. Iadecola C. From CSD to headache: a long and winding road. Nat Med 2002; 8(2):110–2.

21. Koo JW, Balaban CD. Serotonin-induced plasma extravasation in the murine inner ear: possible mechanism of migraine-associated inner ear dysfunction. Cephalalgia 2006;26(11):1310–9.

22. von Brevern M, Zeise D, Neuhauser H, et al. Acute migrainous vertigo: clinical and oculographic findings. Brain 2005;128(Pt 2):365–74.

23. Seemungal BM, Gresty MA, Bronstein AM. The endocrine system, vertigo and balance. Curr Opin Neurol 2001;14(1):27–34.

24. Lopez-Escamez JA, Dlugaiczyk J, Jacobs J, et al. Accompanying symptoms overlap during attacks in Ménière's disease and vestibular migraine. Front Neurol 2014;5:265.

25. Bisdorff A, Von Brevern M, Lempert T, et al. Classification of vestibular symptoms: towards an international classification of vestibular disorders. J Vestib Res 2009; 19(1–2):1–13.

26. Headache Classification Subcommittee of the International Headache Society. The international classification of headache disorders: 2nd edition. Cephalalgia 2004;24(Suppl 1):9–160.

27. Lempert T, Olesen J, Furman J, et al. Vestibular migraine: diagnostic criteria. J Vestib Res 2012;22(4):167–72.

28. Amarenco P, Lévy C, Cohen A, et al. Causes and mechanisms of territorial and nonterritorial cerebellar infarcts in 115 consecutive patients. Stroke 1994;25(1): 105–12.

29. Seemungal BM. Neuro-otological emergencies. Curr Opin Neurol 2007;20(1): 32–9.

30. Newman-Toker DE, Kattah JC, Alvernia JE, et al. Normal head impulse test differentiates acute cerebellar strokes from vestibular neuritis. Neurology 2008;70(24 Pt 2):2378–85.

31. Searls DE, Pazdera L, Korbel E, Vysata O, Caplan LR. Symptoms and signs of posterior circulation ischemia in the new England medical center posterior circulation registry. Arch Neurol 2012;69(3):346–51.

32. Requena T, Espinosa-Sanchez JM, Cabrera S, et al. Familial clustering and genetic heterogeneity in Ménière's disease. Clin Genet 2014;85(3):245–52.

33. Merchant SN, Adams JC, Nadol JB Jr. Pathophysiology of Ménière's syndrome: are symptoms caused by endolymphatic hydrops? Otol Neurotol 2005;26(1):74–81.

34. Harcourt J, Barraclough K, Bronstein AM. Ménière's disease. BMJ 2014;349: g6544.
35. Lopez-Escamez JA, Carey J, Chung WH, et al. Diagnostic criteria for Ménière's disease. J Vest Res 2015;25(1):1–7.
36. Hood JD. Audiological considerations in Ménière's disease. ORL J Otorhinolaryngol Relat Spec 1980;42(1–2):77–90.
37. Carfrae MJ, Holtzman A, Eames F, et al. 3 Tesla delayed contrast magnetic resonance imaging evaluation of Ménière's disease. Laryngoscope 2008;118(3): 501–5.
38. Ge X, Shea JJ Jr. Transtympanic electrocochleography: a 10-year experience. Otol Neurotol 2002;23(5):799–805.
39. Kim HH, Wiet RJ, Battista RA. Trends in the diagnosis and the management of Ménière's disease: results of a survey. Otolaryngol Head Neck Surg 2005; 132(5):722–6.
40. Curthoys IS, Vulovic V, Burgess AM, et al. Neural basis of new clinical vestibular tests: otolithic neural responses to sound and vibration. Clin Exp Pharmacol Physiol 2014;41(5):371–80.
41. Rauch SD, Zhou G, Kujawa SG, et al. Vestibular evoked myogenic potentials show altered tuning in patients with Ménière's disease. Otol Neurotol 2004; 25(3):333–8.
42. Timmer FC, Zhou G, Guinan JJ, et al. Vestibular evoked myogenic potential (VEMP) in patients with Ménière's disease with drop attacks. Laryngoscope 2006;116(5):776–9.
43. Lin MY, Timmer FC, Oriel BS, et al. Vestibular evoked myogenic potentials (VEMP) can detect asymptomatic saccular hydrops. Laryngoscope 2006;116(6):987–92.
44. Park HJ, Migliaccio AA, Della Santina CC, et al. Search-coil head-thrust and caloric tests in Ménière's disease. Acta Otolaryngol 2005;125(8):852–7.
45. Semaan MT, Megerian CA. Ménière's disease: a challenging and relentless disorder. Otolaryngol Clin North Am 2011;44(2):383–403, ix.
46. Huppert D, Strupp M, Brandt T. Long-term course of Ménière's disease revisited. Acta Otolaryngol 2010;130(6):644–51.
47. Thirlwall AS, Kundu S. Diuretics for Ménière's disease or syndrome. Cochrane Database Syst Rev 2006;(3):CD003599.
48. Strupp M, Hupert D, Frenzel C, et al. Long-term prophylactic treatment of attacks of vertigo in Ménière's disease – comparison of a high with a low dosage of betahistine in an open trial. Acta Otolaryngol 2008;128(5):520–4.
49. Gazquez I, Soto-Varela A, Aran I, et al. High prevalence of systemic autoimmune diseases in patients with Menière's disease. PLoS One 2011;6(10):e26759.
50. Boleas-Aguirre MS, Lin FR, Della Santina CC, et al. Longitudinal results with intratympanic dexamethasone in the treatment of Ménière's disease. Otol Neurotol 2008;29(1):33–8.
51. Garduno-Anaya MA, Couthino De Toledo H, Hinojosa-Gonzalez R, et al. Dexamethasone inner ear perfusion by intratympanic injection in unilateral Ménière's disease: a two-year prospective, placebo-controlled, double-blind, randomized trial. Otolaryngol Head Neck Surg 2005;133(2):285–94.
52. Gottshall KR, Hoffer ME, Moore RJ, et al. The role of vestibular rehabilitation in the treatment of Ménière's disease. Otolaryngol Head Neck Surg 2005;133(3): 326–8.

Transient Ischemic Attacks Presenting with Dizziness or Vertigo

Christina A. Blum, MD, Scott E. Kasner, MD*

KEYWORDS

- Posterior circulation • Transient ischemic attack • Vertebrobasilar insufficiency
- Dizziness • Vertigo • Stroke

KEY POINTS

- Transient ischemic attacks (TIAs) and strokes comprise most of the central causes of episodic vestibular syndrome.
- Dizziness with or without associated symptoms is the most common manifestation of posterior circulation TIA.
- The risk of subsequent stroke in patients who are discharged home with a diagnosis of dizziness or vertigo is low.
- Isolated dizziness as a manifestation of posterior circulation TIA is a clinical challenge because most patients are asymptomatic with only normal neurologic examination findings on presentation.
- Large artery atherosclerosis of the vertebrobasilar system is involved in one-third of posterior circulation ischemic events and carries a high early recurrent stroke risk.

CASE SCENARIO

A 65-year-old woman with a history of hypertension and hyperlipidemia presented to the emergency department with 2 episodes of transient vertigo. The first episode occurred 1 week before presentation, and she described it as unprovoked continuous vertigo with nausea that lasted for 5 minutes with subsequent complete resolution. The second episode occurred on the day of presentation and consisted of isolated vertigo associated with nausea and vomiting lasting for 15 minutes. On arrival, she had recovered to her baseline. Her blood pressure was 221/117 mm Hg and her heart rate was 96 beats per minute and regular. Her neurologic examination, including Dix-Hallpike maneuver, was normal. Routine laboratory tests were within normal

Department of Neurology, University of Pennsylvania, 3400 Spruce Street, Philadelphia, PA 19104, USA
* Corresponding author.
E-mail address: kasner@mail.med.upenn.edu

Neurol Clin 33 (2015) 629–642
http://dx.doi.org/10.1016/j.ncl.2015.04.005
0733-8619/15/$ – see front matter © 2015 Elsevier Inc. All rights reserved.

neurologic.theclinics.com

limits. Her ABCD2 (age, blood pressure, clinical features, duration of transient ischemic attack [TIA], and presence of diabetes) score was 3. Electrocardiogram and telemetry showed normal sinus rhythm. MRI showed no evidence of acute infarct. Magnetic resonance angiography (MRA) (**Fig. 1**A) followed by computed tomography angiography (CTA) (see **Fig. 1**B, C) showed intracranial distal vertebral and midbasilar stenosis. She was subsequently admitted for close observation and further evaluation. Lipid panel showed a low-density lipoprotein (LDL) level of 182 mg/dL. Glycosylated hemoglobin (HbA1c) was 7.4%. Echocardiography showed normal ejection fraction, mild left ventricular hypertrophy, and normal left atrial size. The patient was treated with aspirin, antihypertensive medications, statin, and oral hypoglycemic agents and discharged home. One week after discharge, she presented to the emergency department with another transient episode of unprovoked isolated vertigo lasting for 2 minutes. Neurologic examination was again normal. Repeat brain MRI on admission revealed no acute infarct and MRA was unchanged. Clopidogrel was prescribed. The patient's antihypertensive regimen was adjusted and she was discharged home. At 3 months' follow-up, she reported no further events.

INTRODUCTION

TIAs and strokes comprise most of the central causes of episodic vestibular syndrome, although the proportion of patients presenting with dizziness and vertigo to

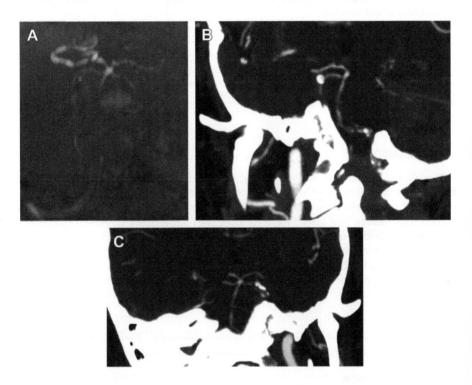

Fig. 1. (A) MRA of the head without contrast showing slow/absent flow in the basilar artery. (B) Computed tomography angiography (CTA) of the head, sagittal projection images, showing severe atherosclerosis in the left vertebral and mid–basilar artery. (C) Coronal CTA of the head showing severe midbasilar stenosis.

emergency departments who turn out to have central causes rather than peripheral causes is small. In contrast, isolated dizziness is a presenting symptom in 10% to 20% of patients with vertebrobasilar ischemia.[1] Multiple studies have shown that dizziness with or without associated neurologic symptoms is the most common symptom of posterior circulation TIA and, most notably, can be more frequent in the days to weeks preceding posterior circulation strokes. It is also well established that this population carries a high risk of subsequent stroke. Isolated dizziness has classically been attributed to benign peripheral causes. It therefore important to recognize isolated dizziness presenting as TIA when it occurs and to appropriately evaluate for underlying TIA mechanism, implement early treatment when indicated, and initiate risk factor modification strategies to prevent recurrent and potentially disabling or fatal ischemic events.

PREVALENCE AND PATHOMECHANISMS

Posterior circulation ischemic events comprise approximately 20% to 25% of all strokes and TIAs.[2] The exact prevalence of TIAs involving the posterior circulation is unknown because the diagnosis of TIA is often based purely on the patient's report of symptoms. Approximately 12% to 18% of patients with a diagnosis of posterior circulation stroke report previous TIA-like symptoms.[3]

Common causes of posterior circulation TIA are large artery atherosclerosis, cardioembolism, and dissection. Large artery atherosclerosis of the vertebrobasilar system is involved in one-third of posterior circulation ischemic events and carries a high annual recurrent stroke risk of 10% to 15% per year.[4–6] Mechanisms of stroke in patients with large artery atherosclerosis involving the posterior circulation include artery-to-artery embolism from an ulcerated plaque in the vertebrobasilar system. Hemodynamic failure may also result from basilar stenosis, severe bilateral vertebral stenosis, or dominant unilateral vertebral stenosis when the contralateral vertebral artery is congenitally hypoplastic. The most common areas of atherosclerotic involvement in the posterior circulation include the distal vertebral arteries at the vertebrobasilar junction, the proximal portion of the vertebral artery, and the proximal to midbasilar artery (**Fig. 2**A). The distribution (intracranial vs extracranial) and location (arterial segment) of atherosclerosis differs by race and gender. Intracranial atherosclerosis is more common in black people, Asians, and women, whereas extracranial atherosclerosis is more common in white people, who also tend to have coexisting carotid, coronary, and peripheral artery disease.[2,7] African American patients may have atherosclerosis in the distal basilar artery, which is also a common site for embolism. Dissection is more likely to occur in the intraforaminal segments of the vertebral artery and the segment between the vertebral foramina and the dura mater.

Vertigo as a symptom is generally thought to result from a pathologic asymmetry of vestibular inputs. Focal stenosis leading to a left-right asymmetry in the vertebrobasilar system can in turn lead to a difference in vestibular input. This difference may occur not only in the setting of atheroembolus but also during a systemic insult; for example, a cardiac arrhythmia leading to systemic hypoperfusion.[8] An additional proposed mechanism explaining the symptom of isolated transient vertigo is a selective vulnerability of the superior labyrinth, which contains the anterior and horizontal semicircular canals and the utricle. The internal auditory artery most commonly arises from the anterior inferior cerebellar artery and divides into the superior branch (anterior vestibular artery) and inferior branch (common cochlear artery) (see **Fig. 2**B). The inferior branch supplies the inferior vestibular labyrinth containing the saccule and posterior

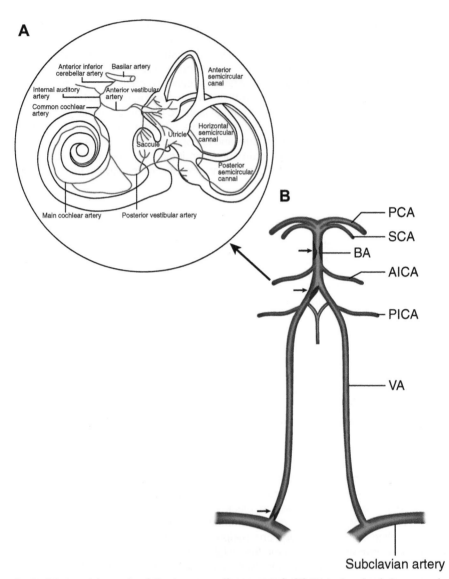

Fig. 2. (*A*) Arterial supply of the inner ear (*large arrow*). (*B*) Posterior circulation vascular anatomy showing common areas affected by atherosclerosis (*small arrows*). AICA, anterior inferior cerebellar artery; BA, basilar artery; PCA, posterior cerebral artery; PICA, posterior inferior cerebellar artery; SCA, superior cerebellar artery; VA, vertebral artery. ([A] *From* Lee H. Audiovestibular loss in anterior inferior cerebellar artery territory infarction: a window to early detection? J Neurol Sci 2012;313:153–9; with permission.)

canal. The common cochlear artery forms anastomoses with the superior branch of the internal auditory artery, which is smaller in caliber and lacks collaterals, thus being most susceptible to flow failure.[9] Other structures commonly implicated in isolated vertigo include the medial branch of the posterior inferior cerebellar artery (PICA), which supplies the cerebellar nodulus; the vestibular nuclei; and the zone of entry of the vestibular nerve (see **Fig. 2**).[2]

Cardioembolism usually involves the PICA, distal basilar artery, superior cerebellar artery, or posterior cerebral artery. Small vessel disease is more commonly associated with posterior circulation strokes rather than TIA and results from either lipohyalinosis or focal atherosclerosis of the small penetrating arteries arising from the intracranial vertebral, basilar, and posterior cerebral arteries. Less common causes of posterior circulation TIA manifesting as transient dizziness include dolichoectasia, subclavian stenosis proximal to the vertebral artery origin, rotational vertebral artery occlusion, fibromuscular dysplasia, and migrainous infarction.

Importantly, anterior circulation ischemia also manifests as dizziness. In a recent systematic review of anterior circulation stroke and TIA manifesting as vestibular syndromes, TIAs were more common than strokes, with the insula, parietal cortex, and adjacent subcortical white matter being the structures most frequently involved. There was a slight preference toward right-sided versus left-sided structures and men versus women.[10]

DEFINITIONS

In this chapter, the terms dizziness and vertigo are used interchangeably in light of past studies that have shown the lack of reliability in patients' description of symptoms, and the lack of any consistent underlying neuroanatomic correlate, pathomechanism, or cause associated with specific symptom descriptors, including dizziness, vertigo, lightheadedness, and unsteadiness.[11] With regard to these vestibular symptoms, which are categorized into one of several vestibular syndromes (discussed elsewhere in this issue), TIA is among the dangerous causes of spontaneous episodic vestibular syndrome.

The most recent American Heart Association/American Stroke Association definition of TIA refers to any transient neurologic deficit presumed to be caused by focal brain, spinal cord, or retinal ischemia without evidence of acute infarction on imaging and lasting less than 24 hours.[12] The previous time-based definition offered an arbitrary definition of TIA as sudden-onset neurologic symptoms lasting less than 24 hours. The tissue-based definition is considered to be more accurate because it takes into account the observation that even brief transient neurologic symptoms (including isolated vertigo[13]) can be associated with infarction on imaging.

Transient neurologic attack (TNA) is a term coined to define any episode of transient neurologic dysfunction. Although TIAs, otherwise known as the dangerous TNAs, signified focal symptoms caused by vascular disorders with a nonfavorable clinical course, TNAs were meant to refer to nonfocal, nonspecific neurologic symptoms (including syncope, confusion, or transient global amnesia) with a more benign clinical course. However, TIAs accompanied by nonfocal symptoms could also portend increased risk of stroke, cardiovascular events, and cognitive impairment.[14,15] Prospective observational studies have shown that dizziness is one of the most common symptoms preceding vertebrobasilar stroke, paralleling amaurosis fugax preceding internal carotid stroke. In spite of this, clinical trials investigating treatment following TIA and stroke have classically excluded patients with isolated dizziness,[16,17] possibly because the number of isolated dizziness presentations attributable to cerebral ischemia is low relative to that of peripheral causes, as is the risk of subsequent stroke in an unselected population of dizzy patients. Thus, patients presenting with transient vertigo might be treated less aggressively than those presenting with focal weakness or speech disturbance, because it may not be possible to generalize these trials to the former population.

DIAGNOSTIC APPROACH: BEDSIDE AND LABORATORY TESTING
History and Examination

When evaluating a patient presenting to the emergency department with transient vertigo, the physician is most often relying on the history alone, because patients are usually asymptomatic by the time of arrival. It is most valuable to ask the patient about the duration of dizziness and possible triggers. Dizziness lasting less than 24 hours classifies the patient under episodic vestibular syndrome and thus guides the subsequent evaluation. Although the presence of vascular risk factors may lower the threshold for more aggressive investigation and treatment, this approach has not been validated and might miss younger patients with ischemia who lack these risk factors. Associated focal symptoms at the time of the episode, including dysarthria, diplopia, dysphagia, hemiataxia, unilateral numbness, or weakness, may indicate a vascular cause; however, approximately 20% of patients experience isolated dizziness. Furthermore, nonfocal symptoms, including imbalance, bilateral weakness, and paresthesias, have been shown to occur with a frequency ranging from 12% to 50% of patients with TIA.[15,18] One study found that nonfocal associated symptoms occurred in 54% of patients in the 6 months preceding a nondisabling stroke or TIA in the posterior circulation, compared with 36% of those involving the anterior circulation.[19] The presence of frank associated neurologic symptoms or craniocervical pain is more likely to be helpful than their absence, because isolated transient vertigo is the most common manifestation of posterior circulation ischemia.

Neurologic examination in patients presenting with spontaneous episodic vestibular syndrome is most often normal. The Dix-Hallpike maneuver may be performed to rule out benign positional vertigo (BPPV), although typically patients with BPPV describe nonspontaneous, positionally triggered symptoms. The HINTS (head impulse, nystagmus, and test for skew) eye movement examination is used to differentiate central from peripheral causes in patients with acute continuous vestibular syndrome.[20] HINTS has limited clinical utility in patients with spontaneous episodic vertigo because these patients are typically asymptomatic with normal eye movements during the evaluation; in occasional patients seen within minutes or hours of onset (whose symptoms abate in <24 hours), HINTS may still prove helpful. Subtle focal examination findings suggestive of a vascular insult may be elicited on careful neurologic examination even in patients who report complete resolution of symptoms. In addition, certain features in the history and examination can help predict subsequent stroke risk in patients with TIA (discussed further later in the article).

Diagnostic Evaluation

Diagnostic evaluation of patients with TIA is extrapolated from existing evidence, because most of the available literature concerns patients with both TIAs and strokes, or stroke alone. Noncontrast head computed tomography (CT) is most sensitive in excluding intracranial hemorrhage and may also show evidence of old infarcts, which may or may not be anatomically relevant to the patient presenting with isolated dizziness. CT is insensitive to acute ischemic stroke[21] and, with posterior circulation ischemia, is additionally susceptible to streak artifact, which may substantially preclude accurate visualization of the posterior fossa. MRI with a diffusion-weighted imaging sequence is most sensitive for evaluating acute ischemic lesions and is more likely to be positive in the case of longer symptom duration and focal neurologic symptoms.[22] However, even MRI is imperfect. Multiple studies have shown that MRI can be falsely negative in up to 20% of clinically definitive posterior circulation strokes when performed within the first 24 to 48 hours.[21,23,24] Particularly in the setting of transient isolated vertigo, diagnosis of underlying posterior circulation ischemia depends more on clinical suspicion than on imaging. It is important to stratify patients presenting with suspected TIA according to risk in order to rapidly and efficiently diagnose and treat the small percentage who have vertebrobasilar disease and, consequently, a higher stroke recurrence rate.

Current guidelines recommend an expedited evaluation including intracranial and extracranial vessel imaging in all patients meeting suspicion.[12] The choice of imaging modality is contingent on resources available at the institution and the presence of potential medical contraindications (eg, the presence of pacemaker precluding MRI or renal failure precluding contrast administration). Although duplex ultrasonography is widely used to evaluate for carotid lesions, it has limited use in detecting stenosis in the vertebral arteries.[25] However, color Doppler shows the direction of flow, which may be reversed in the case of severe vertebrobasilar stenosis or bidirectional in patients with significant subclavian stenosis causing subclavian steal. Similarly, transcranial Doppler shows the direction and velocity of flow in the intracranial portions of the vertebral arteries and the proximal basilar artery. CTA and contrast-enhanced MRA both allow good visualization of the full vertebrobasilar system characterizing the location, degree, and appearance of atherosclerotic disease and are both acceptable options.[25]

Pooled data from 2 prospective studies evaluating patients with TIA and minor stroke with at least 50% vertebrobasilar stenosis suggested that the risk of recurrent vertebrobasilar TIA or stroke is higher in patients with symptomatic vertebrobasilar stenosis than in those without stenosis, with a 3.2-fold higher 90-day risk of recurrent events.[26,27] The risk was highest in the first 30 days and higher for intracranial than extracranial stenosis. It is unclear whether the degree of stenosis in patients with vertebrobasilar ischemia is associated with the risk of recurrent stroke in patients with vertebrobasilar stenosis. Preliminary results from the Vertebrobasilar Flow Evaluation and Risk of Transient Ischaemic Attack and Stroke (VERiTAS) study using software to measure vertebrobasilar flow suggest that flow failure rather than the degree of stenosis is associated with recurrent vertebrobasilar ischemic events in patients with symptomatic vertebrobasilar stenosis.[28]

Cardiac evaluation should be considered in all patients presenting with an episode of isolated dizziness suspected to be TIA, particularly those in whom the mechanism is not suspected to be large artery atherosclerosis. Studies include a 12-lead electrocardiogram (ECG), cardiac monitoring to identify atrial fibrillation, transthoracic echocardiogram (TTE), and transesophageal echocardiogram (TEE) in a subgroup of patients to identify a cardioembolic source. The reported detection rates of new atrial fibrillation on standard ECG or 24-hour telemetry range from 2% to 6% in patients with either stroke or TIA.[29] In the EMBRACE (30-day Cardiac Event Monitor Belt for Recording Atrial fibrillation after a Cerebral Ischemic Event) study, the 30-day detection rate of episodes of atrial fibrillation lasting 30 seconds or longer in patients with cryptogenic TIA was close to 15%.[30] Thus, prolonged cardiac monitoring is useful in detecting paroxysmal atrial fibrillation in patients in sinus rhythm with suspected TIA and no evidence of an alternative cause. These extensive cardiac investigations may be deferred in patients with multiple stereotypical episodes of transient isolated vertigo (without other TIA symptoms), who are unlikely to have a cardioembolic source, because emboli ejected from the heart do not typically go repeatedly to the same vascular territory of the brain.

The yield of an echocardiogram depends on whether there is a clinical evidence of underlying structural heart disease. TTE is noninvasive and best for detecting left ventricular thrombus (especially when done with contrast) and evaluating left ventricular function, particularly in patients with known or suspected heart disease. TEE is superior to TTE in evaluating the left atrial appendage for thrombus or spontaneous echo contrast indicating high thrombotic potential, diagnosing septal defects such as patent foramen ovale, and detecting atheromas of the aortic arch,[31] but is invasive and carries a greater risk of complications from testing. Thus patients with suspected posterior circulation TIA should undergo a TTE, which can then be followed by a TEE in a certain subgroup of patients, particularly in younger patients without heart disease and unknown stroke mechanism after initial evaluation.

Laboratory Tests

Although not systematically validated, initial routine laboratory tests that are generally recommended include complete blood count, comprehensive metabolic panel, coagulation studies, serum biomarkers for acute cardiac disease when clinically suspected (troponin or brain natriuretic peptide), fasting lipid profile, HbA1c, and erythrocyte sedimentation rate. Additional testing, including rapid plasma reagin, blood alcohol level, urine toxicology, blood cultures, and tests for underlying systemic malignancy may be considered depending on the clinical scenario. Hypercoagulability testing may be performed in young patients with otherwise unexplained TIA or stroke, history of unprovoked clots, family history of clotting disorders, or history of spontaneous second-trimester abortion,[12] although there is limited evidence to support the cost-effectiveness and clinical utility of these tests.[32]

ACUTE TREATMENT OPTIONS

Initial management of suspected posterior circulation TIA should consist of the same measures as in ischemic stroke, which are intended to maintain cerebral perfusion and prevent additional impending ischemic injury. Patients with TIA have an increased risk of stroke within 3 months (4%–18.5%) and the risk has been shown to be highest within the first week following TIA.[33]

Routine measures to maintain cerebral perfusion include laying the head of the bed flat during the first 24 hours of onset and administering intravenous (IV) fluids to avoid hypovolemia. Normoglycemia and normothermia should be maintained. Neurologic status should be closely monitored for any change.[34] In the case of a patient with transient symptoms attributable to the posterior circulation who is at high risk of developing a stroke in the first 24 to 48 hours of presentation, early detection of deficits consistent with subsequent stroke while in the hospital can lead to timely treatment with IV tissue plasminogen activator (tPA).

Blood Pressure

Several studies and meta-analyses have shown a U-shaped relationship between baseline or admission systolic blood pressure after TIA/acute stroke and early death, late death, or dependency,[34] although an ideal blood pressure range in the setting of TIA/acute stroke has not been validated. The consensus is that moderate arterial hypertension during acute ischemic stroke might be advantageous by improving cerebral perfusion of the ischemic tissue or tissue at risk. Guidelines recommend not actively treating blood pressure unless it exceeds 220/120 mm Hg. If after 24 hours the patient is clinically stable with no perfusional dependence on neurologic examination, long-term antihypertensive therapy may be initiated.[34]

Medical Therapy

Antithrombotic medications

Current guidelines based on the results of several randomized controlled trials and meta-analyses including patients with TIA and ischemic stroke recommend starting oral aspirin 325 mg within the first 24 to 48 hours to prevent recurrent stroke. Because of the high early risk of stroke after a TIA, several trials are investigating the benefit of short-term dual antiplatelet therapy (30–90 days) in high-risk patients with TIA and minor stroke. The CHANCE (Clopidogrel in High-risk Patients with Acute Non-disabling Cerebrovascular Events) trial, which enrolled 5170 patients within 24 hours after the onset of minor ischemic stroke, evaluated combination therapy with (1) clopidogrel at loading dose of 300 mg followed by 75 mg daily and aspirin 75 mg per day for the first 3 weeks, or (2) aspirin 75 mg per day. The primary outcome was ischemic or hemorrhagic stroke during 90 days of follow-up. Relative risk reduction for stroke with dual antiplatelet therapy compared with aspirin alone was 30% (8.2% vs 11.7%), whereas moderate or severe hemorrhage occurred in 0.3% in each group.[16] Patients with isolated dizziness were excluded from this study, thus limiting the ability to generalize the results to patients with TIA manifesting as transient vertigo. Despite that, there is emerging evidence supporting dual antiplatelet therapy as a short-term strategy in patients with transient vertigo caused by atherosclerotic vertebrobasilar disease.[35] If atrial fibrillation is diagnosed after TIA, anticoagulant therapy rather than antiplatelet therapy should be used in the absence of contraindications.[36]

Statins

In-hospital high-dose statin initiation is one of the mainstays of treatment in all high-risk patients regardless of LDL[36] or in whom the TIA is thought to be caused by large artery atherosclerosis. A prospective observational cohort study involving 7243 patients showed that early statin initiation (defined as in hospital) for patients with TIA significantly reduced recurrent TIA or stroke and did not increase the risk of intracranial hemorrhage.[37] In contrast, intermediate or late initiation (within 1 year or later) resulted in a 49% increase in the composite end point of ischemic stroke, hemorrhagic stroke, TIA, coronary event, or death.[37]

Revascularization

In patients with severe intracranial vertebrobasilar stenosis of 70% to 99%, current evidence from the Stenting versus Aggressive Medical Management for Preventing Recurrent Stroke in Intracranial Stenosis (SAMMPRIS) trial suggests that the 2-year risk of recurrent cerebrovascular events is 2-fold higher in patients undergoing angioplasty and stent placement versus aggressive medical treatment (23% vs 10% respectively).[35] The benefit of extracranial vertebral artery stenting is unclear; however, evidence from retrospective studies suggests low cerebrovascular complication rates and high technical success rates.[38] Given their as-yet unproven safety and efficacy, the use of these devices should be limited to clinical trials. In patients who have recurrent definitive events despite maximal medical therapy and thus were either not included in SAMMPRIS or represented outcome events, procedures can be a consideration, although prospective data on benefit/risk in this setting are limited.

TRIAGE AND DISPOSITION

When a patient presents with a suspected TIA, the decision on whether to admit, observe, or discharge the patient home depends on multiple factors, related to both the clinical picture and the health infrastructure in place. This decision becomes particularly challenging when the only symptom before presentation was transient dizziness and the examination is otherwise normal. The risk of subsequent stroke in patients who are discharged home with a diagnosis of dizziness or vertigo is low (less than 1 in 500) with the risk highest in the first 30 days after discharge.[39] Given the high frequency of emergency department visit discharges with this diagnosis, improving triage and disposition strategies in this patient population is necessary and has the potential to reduce the number of cardiovascular events nationwide. Hospitalization for suspected TIA results in more rapid evaluation for underlying cause, allows for cardiac monitoring, and leads to early implementation of secondary prevention strategies. Some evidence suggests that adherence to treatment is improved if initiated while in the hospital. Early detection of stroke symptoms, should they occur, results in faster treatment with tPA.

The ABCD2 score is a clinical prediction score to help stratify the risk of subsequent stroke in patients presenting with TIA. The components of the ABCD2 score are as follows: age greater than 60 (1 point), blood pressure greater than 140 mm Hg or greater than 90 mm Hg (1 point), symptom characteristics (2 points for motor ± speech, or 1 point for speech), diabetes (1 point), and duration (0 points for <10 minutes, 1 point for 10–59 minutes, 2 points for >60 minutes). Score ranges are divided as 0 to 3, 4 to 5, and 6 to 7, indicating a 1%, 4%, and 8% risk of subsequent stroke in the first 48 hours after TIA, respectively. However, the ABCD2 score does not take into account symptoms suggestive of posterior circulation ischemia, such as vertigo, diplopia, or transient hemifield loss, and patients with isolated vertigo or dizziness were not considered specifically in the development or evaluation of this tool. Another significant limitation in this score is that it does not include results of vessel imaging. Furthermore, several studies attempting to validate the score's use in emergency care settings have shown inconsistent or discouraging results.[40–42] Therefore, although the ABCD2 score may supplement the evaluation of suspected TIA, the utility of this tool in decision making has not been systematically studied and it is not sufficient for triaging patients. Other scores have been more recently developed that may have a better predictive value than the ABCD2 score[43,44] because they include imaging parameters (MRI and vessel imaging) and dual symptoms (ie, similar symptoms in the past week). A drawback of these prediction tools is that they are skewed toward the presence of vascular risk factors, which may be absent in younger populations and in those with other TIA mechanisms such as cervical artery dissection or hypercoagulable states.

In summary, all patients with suspected TIA should undergo appropriate diagnostic evaluation and treatment within 24 hours of presentation, regardless of the setting (hospital, observation unit, outpatient clinic). We suggest that all patients with unprovoked episodic vertigo and evidence of vertebrobasilar stenosis be admitted for expedited evaluation, monitoring, and stroke prevention strategies. If a patient is being discharged home from the emergency room, intracranial and extracranial vessel imaging should be performed expeditiously to exclude symptomatic vertebrobasilar stenosis. Regarding other stroke mechanisms of vertebrobasilar TIAs, investigations regarding approaches that will result in the best clinical outcomes and be most cost-effective are still needed.

Fig. 3 shows a proposed algorithm for triage and disposition of patients with transient dizziness.

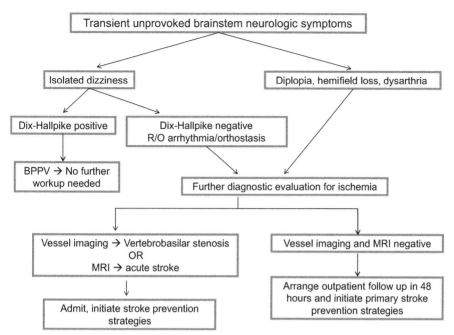

Fig. 3. Suggested algorithm for diagnostic evaluation of patients with transient unprovoked neurologic symptoms.

SUMMARY

Isolated vertigo as a manifestation of posterior circulation TIA is a clinical challenge because most patients on presentation are asymptomatic and have only normal neurologic examination findings. Although it is substantially less common than peripheral causes, posterior circulation ischemia carries a high risk of recurrent events and should be considered as a potential cause of spontaneous episodic vestibular syndrome even in the absence of associated symptoms. Existing tools for risk stratification may not be applicable to patients with transient vertigo. Diagnostic evaluation should include intracranial and extracranial imaging of the vertebral arteries and basilar artery to exclude high-risk conditions such as large artery atherosclerosis, which has a high early stroke recurrence rate. Aggressive medical management with antiplatelet therapy, statin use, and risk factor modification is the mainstay of treatment unless atrial fibrillation is detected, which would prompt anticoagulation. Given the high stroke risk after a TIA in high-risk patients despite current medical therapy, studies designed to improve stroke prevention strategies are underway.

REFERENCES

1. Newman-Toker DE. Diagnosing dizziness in the emergency department: why "what do you mean by 'dizzy'?" Should not be the first question you ask, vol. 3267879. Ann Arbor (MI): ProQuest Information and Learning Company; 2007. p. 220.
2. Markus HS, van der Worp HB, Rothwell PM. Posterior circulation ischaemic stroke and transient ischaemic attack: diagnosis, investigation, and secondary prevention. Lancet Neurol 2013;12:989–98.

3. Paul NL, Simoni M, Rothwell PM. Transient isolated brainstem symptoms preceding posterior circulation stroke: a population-based study. Lancet Neurol 2013;12: 65–71.

4. Qureshi AI, Ziai WC, Yahia AM, et al. Stroke-free survival and its determinants in patients with symptomatic vertebrobasilar stenosis: a multicenter study. Neurosurgery 2003;52:1033–9 [discussion: 1039–40].

5. Prognosis of patients with symptomatic vertebral or basilar artery stenosis. The Warfarin-Aspirin Symptomatic Intracranial Disease (WASID) Study Group. Stroke 1998;29:1389–92.

6. Flossmann E, Rothwell PM. Prognosis of vertebrobasilar transient ischaemic attack and minor stroke. Brain 2003;126:1940–54.

7. Savitz SI, Caplan LR. Vertebrobasilar disease. N Engl J Med 2005;352:2618–26.

8. Newman-Toker DE, Camargo CA Jr. 'Cardiogenic vertigo'–true vertigo as the presenting manifestation of primary cardiac disease. Nat Clin Pract Neurol 2006;2: 167–72 [quiz: 173].

9. Grad A, Baloh RW. Vertigo of vascular origin. Clinical and electronystagmographic features in 84 cases. Arch Neurol 1989;46:281–4.

10. Zhou Y, Lee SH, Mantokoudis G, et al. Vertigo and dizziness in anterior circulation cerebrovascular disease: a systematic review. Neurology 2014;82(10 Suppl): 3.092.

11. Newman-Toker DE, Cannon LM, Stofferahn ME, et al. Imprecision in patient reports of dizziness symptom quality: a cross-sectional study conducted in an acute care setting. Mayo Clin Proc 2007;82:1329–40.

12. Easton JD, Saver JL, Albers GW, et al. Definition and evaluation of transient ischemic attack: a scientific statement for healthcare professionals from the American Heart Association/American Stroke Association Stroke Council; Council on Cardiovascular Surgery and Anesthesia; Council on Cardiovascular Radiology and Intervention; Council on Cardiovascular Nursing; and the Interdisciplinary Council on Peripheral Vascular Disease. The American Academy Of Neurology affirms the value of this statement as an educational tool for neurologists. Stroke 2009;40:2276–93.

13. Schwartz NE, Venkat C, Albers GW. Transient isolated vertigo secondary to an acute stroke of the cerebellar nodulus. Arch Neurol 2007;64:897–8.

14. Hoshino T, Nagao T, Mizuno S, et al. Transient neurological attack before vertebrobasilar stroke. J Neurol Sci 2013;325:39–42.

15. Bos MJ, van Rijn MJ, Witteman JC, et al. Incidence and prognosis of transient neurological attacks. JAMA 2007;298:2877–85.

16. Wang Y, Wang Y, Zhao X, et al. Clopidogrel with aspirin in acute minor stroke or transient ischemic attack. N Engl J Med 2013;369:11–9.

17. Johnston SC, Easton JD, Farrant M, et al. Platelet-oriented Inhibition in New TIA and Minor Ischemic Stroke (POINT) trial: rationale and design. Int J Stroke 2013; 8:479–83.

18. Koudstaal PJ, Algra A, Pop GA, et al. Risk of cardiac events in atypical transient ischaemic attack or minor stroke. The Dutch TIA Study Group. Lancet 1992;340: 630–3.

19. Compter A, Kappelle LJ, Algra A, et al. Nonfocal symptoms are more frequent in patients with vertebral artery than carotid artery stenosis. Cerebrovasc Dis 2013; 35:378–84.

20. Kattah JC, Talkad AV, Wang DZ, et al. Hints to diagnose stroke in the acute vestibular syndrome: Three-step bedside oculomotor examination more sensitive than early MRI diffusion-weighted imaging. Stroke 2009;40:3504–10.

21. Chalela JA, Kidwell CS, Nentwich LM, et al. Magnetic resonance imaging and computed tomography in emergency assessment of patients with suspected acute stroke: a prospective comparison. Lancet 2007;369:293–8.
22. Crisostomo RA, Garcia MM, Tong DC. Detection of diffusion-weighted MRI abnormalities in patients with transient ischemic attack: correlation with clinical characteristics. Stroke 2003;34:932–7.
23. Oppenheim C, Stanescu R, Dormont D, et al. False-negative diffusion-weighted MR findings in acute ischemic stroke. AJNR Am J Neuroradiol 2000;21: 1434–40.
24. Tarnutzer AA, Berkowitz AL, Robinson KA, et al. Does my dizzy patient have a stroke? A systematic review of bedside diagnosis in acute vestibular syndrome. CMAJ 2011;183:E571–92.
25. Khan S, Cloud GC, Kerry S, et al. Imaging of vertebral artery stenosis: a systematic review. J Neurol Neurosurg Psychiatry 2007;78:1218–25.
26. Gulli G, Khan S, Markus HS. Vertebrobasilar stenosis predicts high early recurrent stroke risk in posterior circulation stroke and TIA. Stroke 2009;40:2732–7.
27. Marquardt L, Kuker W, Chandratheva A, et al. Incidence and prognosis of > or = 50% symptomatic vertebral or basilar artery stenosis: Prospective population-based study. Brain 2009;132:982–8.
28. Amin-Hanjani S, Rose-Finnell L, Richardson D, et al. Vertebrobasilar Flow Evaluation and Risk of Transient Ischaemic Attack and Stroke Study (VERITAS): rationale and design. Int J Stroke 2010;5:499–505.
29. Kishore A, Vail A, Majid A, et al. Detection of atrial fibrillation after ischemic stroke or transient ischemic attack: a systematic review and meta-analysis. Stroke 2014; 45:520–6.
30. Gladstone DJ, Spring M, Dorian P, et al. Atrial fibrillation in patients with cryptogenic stroke. N Engl J Med 2014;370:2467–77.
31. de Bruijn SF, Agema WR, Lammers GJ, et al. Transesophageal echocardiography is superior to transthoracic echocardiography in management of patients of any age with transient ischemic attack or stroke. Stroke 2006;37:2531–4.
32. Morris JG, Singh S, Fisher M. Testing for inherited thrombophilias in arterial stroke: Can it cause more harm than good? Stroke 2010;41:2985–90.
33. Kerber KA, Zahuranec DB, Brown DL, et al. Stroke risk after nonstroke emergency department dizziness presentations: a population-based cohort study. Ann Neurol 2014;75:899–907.
34. Jauch EC, Saver JL, Adams HP Jr, et al. Guidelines for the early management of patients with acute ischemic stroke: a guideline for healthcare professionals from the American Heart Association/American Stroke Association. Stroke 2013;44: 870–947.
35. Derdeyn CP, Chimowitz MI, Lynn MJ, et al. Aggressive medical treatment with or without stenting in high-risk patients with intracranial artery stenosis (SAMMPRIS): the final results of a randomised trial. Lancet 2014;383:333–41.
36. Kernan WN, Ovbiagele B, Black HR, et al. Guidelines for the prevention of stroke in patients with stroke and transient ischemic attack: a guideline for healthcare professionals from the American Heart Association/American Stroke Association. Stroke 2014;45:2160–236.
37. Chen PS, Cheng CL, Kao Yang YH, et al. Impact of early statin therapy in patients with ischemic stroke or transient ischemic attack. Acta Neurol Scand 2014;129: 41–8.
38. Radak D, Babic S, Sagic D, et al. Endovascular treatment of symptomatic high-grade vertebral artery stenosis. J Vasc Surg 2014;60:92–7.

39. Kim AS, Fullerton HJ, Johnston SC. Risk of vascular events in emergency department patients discharged home with diagnosis of dizziness or vertigo. Ann Emerg Med 2011;57:34–41.

40. Perry JJ, Sharma M, Sivilotti ML, et al. Prospective validation of the ABCD2 score for patients in the emergency department with transient ischemic attack. CMAJ 2011;183:1137–45.

41. Amarenco P, Labreuche J, Lavallee PC. Patients with transient ischemic attack with ABCD2 <4 can have similar 90-day stroke risk as patients with transient ischemic attack with ABCD2 ≥4. Stroke 2012;43:863–5.

42. Purroy F, Jimenez-Caballero PE, Mauri-Capdevila G, et al. Predictive value of brain and vascular imaging including intracranial vessels in transient ischaemic attack patients: external validation of the ABCD3-I score. Eur J Neurol 2013;20: 1088–93.

43. Merwick A, Albers GW, Amarenco P, et al. Addition of brain and carotid imaging to the ABCD(2) score to identify patients at early risk of stroke after transient ischaemic attack: a multicentre observational study. Lancet Neurol 2010;9:1060–9.

44. Song B, Fang H, Zhao L, et al. Validation of the ABCD3-I score to predict stroke risk after transient ischemic attack. Stroke 2013;44:1244–8.

Medical and Psychiatric Causes of Episodic Vestibular Symptoms

William J. Meurer, MD, MS[a,b],*, Phillip A. Low, MD[c], Jeffrey P. Staab, MD, MS[d]

KEYWORDS

- Episodic vestibular symptoms • Orthostasis • Panic disorders
- Medication adverse effects • Syncope • Dizziness • Vertigo

KEY POINTS

- Episodic dizziness and vertigo symptoms present a diagnostic and therapeutic challenge.
- When taking a history from a patient with episodic dizziness symptoms, a comprehensive discussion regarding associated symptoms and potential alleviating or aggravating factors is crucial because it is the pattern of symptoms together, rather than the nature of individual symptoms alone, that is crucial for differential diagnosis.
- After specific structural/vestibular causes are ruled out by history, physical examination, and other appropriate diagnostic testing, it is reasonable to consider causes such as orthostatic dizziness, postural orthostatic tachycardia syndrome, presyncope, and panic attacks as fully or partially explaining the episodes.

CASE SCENARIO

A 72-year-old woman presents to the emergency department with episodic dizziness at approximately noon. She cannot identify any provoking factors. The episodes have been occurring for some time, at least for the past several months, and occur with varying frequency, sometimes daily, other times, weekly. At times, she feels a lack of balance during these episodes, but has never fallen or lost consciousness. She is not sure if she has noticed any associated spinning sensations during the episodes. She reports that the episodes vary in intensity ranging from a minor irritant to intensely

[a] Department of Emergency Medicine, University of Michigan, Taubman Center B1-354 SPC 5303, 1500 East Medical Center Drive, Ann Arbor, MI 48109, USA; [b] Department of Neurology, University of Michigan, Taubman Center B1-354 SPC 5303, 1500 East Medical Center Drive, Ann Arbor, MI 48109, USA; [c] Department of Neurology, Mayo Clinic, 200 First Street SW, Rochester, MN 55905, USA; [d] Department of Psychiatry and Psychology, Mayo Clinic, 200 First Street SW, Rochester, MN 55905, USA
* Corresponding author. Department of Emergency Medicine, University of Michigan, Taubman Center B1-354 SPC 5303, 1500 East Medical Center Drive, Ann Arbor, MI 48109.
E-mail address: wmeurer@med.umich.edu

Neurol Clin 33 (2015) 643–659
http://dx.doi.org/10.1016/j.ncl.2015.04.007
0733-8619/15/$ – see front matter © 2015 Elsevier Inc. All rights reserved.

distressing. The symptoms are present currently, yet mild in intensity, and she first noticed them today after completing breakfast. The dizziness is occasionally associated with headache and at other times nausea. She denies a history of migraines and current headache, focal weakness, numbness, nausea, or other recent illness. She reports a past medical history of hypertension, transient ischemic attack (TIA), coronary artery disease, fibromyalgia, anxiety, and colonic diverticulosis. Her current medications include lisinopril, gabapentin, aspirin, metoprolol, and atorvastatin, and there have been no recent changes in these medications. She denies the use of alcohol, tobacco, or illicit drugs and lives with her husband, who has mild cognitive impairment. Her family history is negative for stroke or central nervous system malignancy. Her complaint of dizziness persists. On physical examination, her pulse is 72, and respirations 16, blood pressure 133/74, temperature 37.0°C, and pulse oximetry 99% on room air. The blood pressure is repeated while sitting and standing and she has a 23-mm Hg drop in her systolic pressure. Her symptom intensity does not change at all during the orthostatic check. Her general medical examination is entirely within normal limits, and her cardiac examination specifically reveals normal S1 and S2, along with the absence of murmurs, rubs, and gallops. On neurologic examination, her mental status reveals she is oriented to place, person, time, and situation and conversant. On cranial nerve testing, she has normal pupillary responses; her visual fields are full to confrontation, and she has normal facial strength, normal speech, and normal facial sensation. Her extraocular movements are intact and she has no spontaneous or gaze-evoked nystagmus or skew deviation. She has 5/5 strength proximally and distally in both upper and lower extremities; sensation is intact to pinprick throughout all modalities tested. Deep tendon reflexes are 2/2 in the upper and lower extremities. Finger-to-nose and heel-to-shin testing is accurate. Casual gait is tested and intact. Dix-Hallpike testing does not provoke any nystagmus or symptoms. She is placed on a cardiac monitor and normal sinus rhythm without ectopy is observed. An intravenous line is inserted and blood tests are sent to the laboratory. Her complete blood count, renal function, hepatic function, thyroid function, and urinalysis are normal. A 12-lead electrocardiogram is obtained and is normal. Her symptoms slowly start to improve, although they do not resolve completely, and she requests discharge to home. Her husband presents to the room from their house; however, the nurse is uncomfortable discharging the patient to him, because he is extremely confused. The patient reports to you that this is atypical, and he normally can attend to all activities of daily living and converse quite fluently. You have the husband registered as a patient; his examination reveals no focal deficits, but he and his wife report he has had new-onset headaches over the past 6 weeks. Blood co-oximetry obtained from husband and wife confirms an elevated carbon monoxide level. The fire department goes to the home and finds a malfunctioning furnace. After 4 hours on oxygen by high-flow mask, both patients have returned to baseline, and the husband's headache and wife's dizziness have completely resolved.

INTRODUCTION

Dizziness and vertigo are among the most common presenting patient complaints in ambulatory settings. Specific vestibular causes are often not immediately identifiable. The focus of this article is the potential causes of episodic dizziness and vertigo from other medical and psychiatric conditions. A general approach for arriving at the more specific and potentially more serious causes is provided in other sections of this issue addressing those disorders. The important vestibular causes of episodic dizziness and vertigo include benign paroxysmal positional vertigo (BPPV), vestibular migraine, and

Meniere disease. An important, yet challenging cerebrovascular cause is TIA. The first task of the clinician is to attempt to rule in the above disorders through history taking, physical examination, and diagnostic testing. Many patients with dizziness and vertigo are unable to be diagnosed with the above conditions. As with any undifferentiated patient, the focus in this setting is to attempt to identify the cause that requires urgent attention. Important considerations include orthostatic dizziness (OD), presyncope, medication effects, metabolic causes such as hypoglycemia, anxiety disorders, hyperventilation, and perhaps cervical degenerative spine disease. With the exception of hypoglycemia, the front-line clinician will be challenged to make definitive diagnoses of any of these conditions and may need to refer the patient for additional testing. This review on medical and psychiatric causes is structured by describing a general approach, and then specific historical, physical examination, and diagnostic considerations for the major potential nonvestibular causes of episodic dizziness.

DEFINITIONS

The international nomenclature published by the Bárány Society in 2009 defined vertigo as a sensation of motion (eg, spinning, tilting, translating) when none is present, unsteadiness as a sensation of swaying or rocking when upright, and dizziness as a nonmotion sensation of disturbed spatial orientation.[1] Collectively, these are considered vestibular symptoms. Lightheadedness was not defined by the Bárány Society as a vestibular symptom and was described as a swooning or presyncopal sensation. As patients may not be easily or reliably classified into these symptom clusters, the general term dizziness is used to encapsulate lightheadedness, vestibular symptoms, and other sensations of disequilibrium or unsteadiness. When referring more specifically to the more precise definition of dizziness as a nonmotion sensation, the term vestibular dizziness is used.

EPIDEMIOLOGY

Episodic dizziness is common in the general population, and clear, specific presentations of discrete diseases like BPPV represent a relative minority of cases. Many patients do not seek care with a physician. A population-based, cross-sectional study of a nationally representative sample of 4869 Germans found the annual prevalence of dizziness or vertigo of 22.9%. A subset underwent detailed neuro-otologic evaluations, and the prevalence of vestibular causes was 4.8% of the population; in addition, more than half of subjects with vestibular causes reported additional nonvestibular diagnoses.[2] An additional population-based study in France found that although only 5% of the population had received a specific vestibular diagnosis, the 1-year prevalence is quite high for vertigo (49.3%), unsteadiness (39.1%), and dizziness (35.6%). This symptom-based study also found strong correlation between vertigo and dizziness symptoms and migraines, motion sickness susceptibility, anxiety/depression, and vasovagal episodes.[3]

BEDSIDE DIAGNOSIS

As previously mentioned, the key is to exclude readily identifiable causes like BPPV. Although early clinical training in medicine emphasizes the importance of a thorough history and physical examination when constructing a differential diagnosis for a new complaint, one must recognize the limitations of patients as storytellers and clinicians as listeners.[4] As such, an overreliance on classification by symptom character is problematic.[5] Careful history taking regarding the timing and context of events, along with a physical examination capable of detecting subtle neurologic deficits, can help the clinician overcome the limitations conferred by symptom description.

History

In several textbooks and other commonly used reference materials accessed by front-line medical providers, the traditional focus on history taking for patients with dizziness is to attempt to get the patient to classify the sensation, especially as spinning or not spinning.[6–10] In addition, electronic resources are an increasing tool both in physician training and in medical practice and one specific tool was demonstrated to be associated with improved hospital level outcomes.[11] Examination of this tool found that the approach to vertigo chapter advocated the more traditional approach, whereas the approach to dizziness chapter recognized that this traditional approach leads to frequent misclassification of patients given the vagaries of this challenging symptoms presentation.[5,12–15] Despite the challenges induced by difficulty in symptom description and characterization, one should not undervalue other aspects of the history. When considering episodic dizziness, a comprehensive discussion regarding associated symptoms and potential alleviating or aggravating factors is extremely important. It is the patterns of symptoms together, rather than the nature of individual symptoms alone, that are crucial for differential diagnosis. The timing of episodes may help provide insight into specific nonotologic causes—this includes the frequency, duration, and context—both the timing and any obvious triggers of the symptoms. In addition, history taking should focus on recent changes in medications or medication levels (worsening renal insufficiency) along with other exposures. Many patients with dizziness will have concurrent headache, and one should attempt to establish the degree of temporal correlation between the dizziness symptoms and the head pain; the general discussion here focuses more on situations where the headache is unrelated to the dizziness. Clearly, challenges exist in determining the primary symptom when considering patients with coexisting headaches. The general rule that one should not rely too heavily on detailed characterization of individual vestibular symptoms alone is also well applied to headache and nausea.

Physical Examination

A comprehensive general medical examination and focused neurologic examination are important. A general decline in the rigor of physical examination has been observed for decades in medical care, because diagnostic testing has become increasingly available and relied on.[16] Clearly, this is of particular concern in the evaluation of the patient with nonspecific vestibular symptoms or lightheadedness because both the characterization of the main symptom sensation and the routine diagnostic testing are often unreliable, making a careful physical examination all the more important in these cases.

For the purposes of this review, it is assumed that a thorough and appropriate examination has been conducted and no specific findings implicating a vestibular disorder or newly acquired neurologic deficit have been found. The careful clinician should look for nystagmus in neutral gaze, along with gaze-evoked nystagmus. In patients with episodic, positionally provoked dizziness, a Dix-Hallpike test is an essential part of the examination. The history may not be reliable enough to establish a positional trigger; therefore, the Dix-Hallpike test is an important part of the physical examination of patients with episodic vestibular symptoms. In addition, subtle cranial nerve findings, such as visual field deficits, facial hemi-anesthesia, subtle dysarthria, or tongue deviation, should be excluded through careful examination because small posterior circulation strokes may present with relatively limited examination findings. Younger patients with posterior circulation stroke are particularly at risk for delayed diagnosis.[17] Especially in the emergency department setting, gait testing is important to exclude central cerebellar lesions that may not cause abnormalities in typical bedside coordination testing.

Initial Management and Further Diagnostic Testing

Although cardiac evaluation is generally considered to be of low yield in patients with isolated dizziness, a surprisingly large proportion of patients with acute heart disease and dizziness present with symptoms of vertigo. One should avoid the approach of deferring a cardiac evaluation simply because the patient reports a spinning sensation given the relatively high prevalence of findings in this group.[14] Although the discussion of the risk stratification of potential acute coronary syndromes in the emergency department is beyond the scope of this review, it is reasonable to obtain a 12-lead electrocardiogram and in certain cases obtain continuous cardiac monitoring.[18] Additional blood testing to exclude other obvious causes, such as anemia, hypoglycemia, or dehydration, is reasonable, although it is important to note that such testing is of extremely low value if a positive diagnosis of a vestibular cause such as BPPV is established via positional testing. The degree to which TIA is excluded by the history and physical examination is an additional area that requires careful consideration and is covered in a separate article in this issue.

SPECIFIC CONDITIONS THAT CAN CAUSE EPISODIC DIZZINESS

In the next section, several specific conditions that ultimately are implicated in causing symptomatic, episodic dizziness are considered. Briefly reviewed is the epidemiology of each, along with historical and physical findings that may suggest these conditions. It is important to recognize that many of these conditions cannot be ruled in definitively and may overlap.

Orthostatic Hypotension

Orthostatic hypotension (OH) is defined as a 20-mm Hg drop in systolic blood pressure or a 10-mm Hg drop in diastolic blood pressure within 3 minutes of standing; a subtype known as initial OH occurs a few seconds after standing.[19] A population-based study in Germany using validated neuro-otologic methods and trained interviewers found the 1-year prevalence of OD was approximately 10%.[20] This study used the following criteria to define OD:

- Nonvestibular dizziness (ie, diffuse nonrotational dizziness, lightheadedness, feeling of impending black out or faint) is the most common symptom[21]
- Provocation by postural changes on standing up from a supine or sitting position
- Duration of symptoms seconds to a maximum of 5 minutes
- The absence of vestibular vertigo as defined by the validated study criteria (ie, absence of rotational vertigo, positional vertigo, or recurrent dizziness with nausea and either oscillopsia or episodic imbalance).

A bimodal distribution for age was observed, with the greatest prevalence in young adults and older adults. OD was about 1.6 times more likely in women. OD constituted more than half of subjects with nonvestibular dizziness, the commonest type identified by the study. Illustrating the substantial personal impact exerted by nonvestibular OD, about 18% of the OD cohort from the German study had experienced a fall, with about one-third of the falls resulting in trauma; a third had a fear of falling.[20] Not surprisingly because of the potential for dysautonomia, both OH and OD are more common in adult diabetics.[22]

Some populations are particularly at risk for OD, which has been reported as associated with war victims, dating back to the US Civil War, along with more contemporary references to posttraumatic stress disorder.[23,24] Previous reports have found Asian populations are particularly at risk for measurable orthostasis, and the syndrome of dizziness- and palpitation-predominant orthostatic panic has been reported in Cambodians.[25] Genetic polymorphisms may contribute to OH susceptibility along a biologically plausible autonomic mechanism. A cohort study in China focused on adults with untreated hypertension found that 8.4% of OH subjects had the β1-adrenergic receptor Arg389/Gly polymorphism, relative to 4.2% of non-OH subjects.[26] Consistent with the general epidemiology of OH, this association was stronger for women.

A direct relationship between OH and vestibular dysfunction was demonstrated in a recent case series; rotatory vertigo was induced by presumed generalized cerebral hypoperfusion during OH.[27] Several patterns of nystagmus were observed in about one-third of the patients during induced OH, including downbeat, torsional, and horizontal. Patients with longer durations of orthostatic intolerance had a higher likelihood of developing nystagmus and rotatory vertigo.

In summary, OD may be supported by historical findings and possibly be reproducible in the clinical setting. Referral for autonomic testing can be considered in more obscure cases. Given the overall high prevalence of OH, especially among older adults, a careful consideration of other causes should precede the attribution of episodic dizziness to OD.

Postural Tachycardia Syndrome

Orthostatic intolerance occurs in patients with neurogenic OH (see above discussion), postural tachycardia syndrome (POTS), and reflex syncope (vasovagal and vasodepressor syncope). POTS is defined as the development of symptoms of orthostatic intolerance (including dizziness) associated with an orthostatic heart rate increment of greater than 30 bpm. The condition is common, occurring about 5 to 10 times as frequently as OH.[28–30] Patients with POTS also have an increased risk of developing reflex syncope, and the most common symptoms are lightheadedness, dizziness, nausea, palpitations, and tremulousness.[29] Pathophysiologically, major mechanisms are hypovolemia, deconditioning, and somatic hypervigilance.[30,31] Patients with chronic fatigue and fibromyalgia (see later discussion) are commonly associated with POTS.[32] The diagnosis of POTS is made by autonomic studies to rule out autonomic failure and to record orthostatic tachycardia and the reproduction of orthostatic symptoms. The orthostatic intolerance in POTS is sustained and should be distinguished from the transient dizziness, occurring in when an otherwise normal subject stands up quickly and has transient lightheadedness. On autonomic testing, there is an abrupt, often marked decrease in blood pressure occurring in the first minute with rapid recovery. These patients have normal baroreflexes and do not have autonomic failure. The mechanism is suspected to be due to venous pooling. Of course, this benign condition needs to be distinguished from the autonomic neuropathies.

SYNCOPE/PRESYNCOPE (ARRHYTHMIA/NEUTRALLY MEDIATED SYNCOPE)

Patients with overt loss of consciousness should undergo evaluation for structural cause of syncope.[33] The Choosing Wisely items contributed by the American College of Emergency Physicians recommend against any imaging when the neurologic examination is normal. In patients with syncope or presyncope, perhaps the most serious considerations are vertebrobasilar disease and malignant cardiac arrhythmias;

vertebrobasilar disease is generally not a major consideration in the absence of other unexplained neurologic signs or symptoms plausibly referable to the brain or brainstem. Many patients have less obvious presentations and in those without overt syncope, a consideration of the general causes of neutrally mediated and other forms of syncope is useful for patients with lightheadedness (**Box 1**). It is important to recognize that the same list of causes of syncope cause near-syncope, and the potential for adverse outcomes seems similar in patients with syncope or near-syncope.[34]

Lightheadedness seems to vary throughout the menstrual cycle, and this variation does not seem modified by a past history of vasovagal episodes.[35] In women of child-bearing age, it may be useful to assess for relatedness to menses.

Some cases demonstrate interesting potential concurrent diagnoses. In one case, the head-impulse test precipitated vagally mediated complete heart block in a patient with a recent, pre-existing peripheral vertigo presentation.[36] In another case, a patient initially diagnosed with paroxysmal positional vertigo was finally noted to have neurally mediated presyncope secondary to bradycardia on a longer-term event monitor despite initial extensive neurology and cardiology evaluations.[37] The patient exhibited an intense fear of turning onto his right side, and therefore, positional testing never provoked nystagmus. Ultimately, his symptoms resolved after placement of a cardiac pacemaker. Autonomic dizziness is a consideration when other structural causes are excluded. Specialized testing, including hypercarbic challenge, was able to better confirm autonomic dysfunction in many patients at a tertiary dizziness clinic because standard autonomic testing is often normal.[38]

MEDICATION EFFECTS

In general, medications are most likely to cause dizziness when first started, although abrupt withdrawal may cause dizziness in some cases. The new medication may exert the effect directly, or changes in the metabolism of a different, pre-existing medication may be induced leading to symptoms. In addition, worsening hepatic or renal function may change medication clearance. Even when symptoms seem to be temporally related to a new medication, it is prudent to ensure specific vestibular and serious central causes of dizziness have been considered and reasonably excluded. In certain cases, the drug effect may also induce a physiologic change to better solidify the diagnosis (ie, decreased clearance of a β-blocker leading to dizziness associated with worsened bradycardia).

Dizziness and vertigo comprised 5% of all adverse drug reactions reported in an Italian pharmacovigilance study.[39] Anticonvulsants, antihypertensives, antibiotics, antidepressants, antipsychotics, and anti-inflammatories were most commonly reported. Although these medications are used by a large proportion of the population, these classes have potential actions on the central nervous, autonomic, or cardiovascular systems that likely induce lightheadedness, dizziness, or vertigo. Abruptly stopping antidepressants may cause an antidepressant discontinuation syndrome that includes vestibular symptoms. Dizziness is the most common symptom of sudden withdrawal from selective serotonin uptake inhibitors and serotonin norepinephrine reuptake inhibitors. Withdrawal from tricyclic antidepressants may include vertigo and ataxia. Additional somatic, gastrointestinal, and psychiatric symptoms are likely to manifest themselves on sudden withdrawal from most antidepressants.[40] Dietary supplements and herbal treatments are associated with reported dizziness, although limited by the self-reported nature of nutrition studies; ginkgo biloba has been implicated as perhaps the agent most frequently inducing dizziness.[41]

Box 1
Classification of syncope

Reflex (neutrally mediated) syncope

Vasovagal:

- Mediated by emotional distress: fear, pain, instrumentation, blood phobia
- Mediated by orthostatic stress

Situational:

- Cough, sneeze
- Gastrointestinal stimulation (swallow, defacation, visceral pain)
- Micturition (after micturition)
- After exercise
- After prandial
- Others (eg, laughter, brass instrument playing, weight-lifting)

Carotid sinus syncope

Atypical forms (without apparent triggers or atypical presentation)

Syncope due to orthostatic hypotension

Primary autonomic failure:

- Pure autonomic failure, multiple system atrophy, Parkinson disease with autonomic failure, Lewy body dementia

Secondary autonomic failure:

- Diabetes, amyloidosis, uremia, spinal cord injuries

Drug-induced orthostatic hypotension:

- Alcohol, vasodilators, diuretics, phenothiazines, antidepressants

Volume depletion:

- Hemorrhage, diarrhea, vomiting, other

Cardiac syncope (cardiovascular)

Arrhythmia as primary cause:

  Bradycardia:

- Sinus node dysfunction (including bradycardia/tachycardia syndrome)
- Atrioventricular conduction system disease
- Implanted device malfunction

  Tachycardia:

- Supraventricular
- Ventricular (idiopathic, secondary to structural heart disease or to channelopathies)

  Drug-induced bradycardia and tachyarrhythmias

Structural disease:

  Cardiac: cardiac valvular disease, acute myocardial infarction/ischemia, hypertrophic cardiomyopathy, cardiac masses (atrial myxoma, tumors), pericardial disease/tamponade, congenital anomalies of coronary arteries, prosthetic valves dysfunction

  Others: pulmonary embolus, acute aortic dissection, pulmonary hypertension

From Moya A, Sutton R, Ammirati F, et al. Guidelines for the diagnosis and management of syncope (version 2009). The Task Force for the Diagnosis and Management of Syncope of the European Society of Cardiology (ESC). Eur Heart J 2009;30:2636. Available at: http://eurheartj.oxfordjournals.org/ehj/30/21/2631.full.pdf [Table 4]; with permission.

HYPOGLYCEMIA AND TOXIC/METABOLIC CAUSES

Acute symptomatic hypoglycemia may cause sensations of dizziness or vertigo, although typically this cause is found in patients receiving insulin or other glucose-modulating medications. In less obvious cases, suspected to be metabolic in origin, disorders causing hypoinsulinemia or hyperinsulinemia can be found.[42] A variety of other metabolic causes may contribute to dizziness, and testing for glucose tolerance, thyroid function, and lipid metabolism may be reasonable in cases where a metabolic cause is suspected.[43] A temporal relationship to hypoglycemia (or other metabolic derangements) confirmed by blood testing should be established to attribute episodic dizziness to this cause.

Carbon monoxide is the great mimicker and can lead to both acute and chronic neurologic symptoms, with dizziness and headache being prominent.[44,45] As in the case discussed above, consideration of carbon monoxide poisoning is suggested by vague neurologic symptoms in multiple individuals residing in a location. Many individuals live alone, so a history of symptom resolution while in the school or workplace (or alternative for workplace exposures, in the home) can provide clues to this potential cause as well.

Although becoming less common because of fortification of food products, thiamine deficiency is an important cause of dizziness. Generally, one would expect thiamine deficiency to elicit more ongoing rather than transient symptoms along with eye movement abnormalities. Despite this, if the history suggests the possibility of malnutrition or focal malabsorption (ie, gastric bypass), it is reasonable to initiate supplementation and check serum levels.

VISUAL DISORDERS

The close relationship between the vestibular and visual systems requires consideration of potential visual causes of episodic dizziness or vertigo.[46] Oscillopsia is an illusion of movement in one's visual surroundings; just as with patients having difficulty characterizing dizziness, those with oscillopsia may endorse "blurry vision," "wobbly," and "shimmering." Oscillopsia is much more likely to be a symptom of bilateral peripheral or central vestibular disorders than general medical conditions. In contrast, patients with visually induced dizziness (visual vertigo) may develop dizziness or imbalance in certain visual environments that are busy, such as supermarkets. Visually induced dizziness may be the sequela of previous acute vestibular, neurologic, general medical, or psychiatric disorders. It tends to be more chronic than episodic and may occur alone or as one symptom of persistent postural-perceptual dizziness (PPPD; see later discussion). Patients with visually induced dizziness often avoid provocative situations, giving an appearance of agoraphobia.[47]

CERVICAL SPONDYLOSIS

The data are conflicting regarding an independent relationship between structural spine disease in the neck and dizziness. An observational study of 91 patients with different grades of cervical spine degeneration found that there was no correlation with changes in flow volume in the vertebral arteries and the presence of vertigo.[48] A more recent study investigating patients both with and without vertigo and with and without cervical spondylosis found markedly decreased vertebral artery flow with a 60° rotation in the vertigo-positive, cervical spondylosis patients relative to the vertigo-negative, non-spondylosis patients. In addition, higher burden of spondylosis was significantly associated with decreased vertebral artery flow with neck rotation.[49] Clearly, in cases of transient vertebral artery insufficiency induced by degenerative spinal changes, episodic dizziness should only be associated with neck rotation.

PANIC ATTACKS AND ANXIETY DISORDERS

Panic attacks frequently cause dizziness, lightheadedness, and unsteadiness. In fact, these vestibular symptoms are second only to cardiopulmonary symptoms (eg, chest pain, dyspnea) as common manifestations of panic attacks. Vertigo occurs infrequently with panic attacks and is generally less dramatic than the spinning sensations caused by acute peripheral vestibular disorders. Panic attacks can be recognized by the characteristic symptoms listed in **Box 2**.[50] They have a rapid onset within minutes

---

Box 2
Diagnostic criteria for panic attacks from Diagnostic and Statistical Manual of Mental Disorders 5

A. Recurrent unexpected panic attacks. A panic attack is an abrupt surge of intense fear or intense discomfort that reaches a peak within minutes, during which time 4 (or more) of the following symptoms occur:

 1. Palpitations, pounding heart, or accelerated heart rate

 2. Sweating

 3. Trembling or shaking

 4. Sensations of shortness of breath or smothering

 5. Feelings of choking

 6. Chest pain or discomfort

 7. Nausea or abdominal distress

 8. Feeling dizzy, unsteady, light-headed, or faint

 9. Chills or heat sensations

 10. Paresthesias (numbness or tingling sensations)

 11. Derealization (feelings of unreality) or depersonalization (being detached from oneself)

 12. Fear of losing control or "going crazy"

 13. Fear of dying

B. At least one of the attacks has been followed by 1 mo (or more) of one or both of the following:

 1. Persistent concern or worry about additional panic attacks or their consequences (eg, losing control, having a heart attack, "going crazy")

 2. A significant maladaptive change in behavior related to the attacks (eg, behaviors designed to avoid having panic attacks, such as avoidance of exercise or unfamiliar situations)

C. The disturbance is not attributable to the physiologic effects of a substance (eg, a drug of abuse, a medication) or another medical condition (eg, hyperthyroidism, cardiopulmonary disorders)

D. The disturbance is not better explained by another mental disorder (eg, the panic attacks do not occur only in response to feared social situations, as in social anxiety disorder; in response to circumscribed phobic objects or situations, as in specific phobia; in response to obsessions, as in obsessive-compulsive disorder; in response to reminders of traumatic events, as in posttraumatic stress disorder; or in response to separation from attachment figures, as in separation anxiety disorder).

and may occur spontaneously or be triggered by stimuli that the patient recognizes as fear-provoking. Panic attacks are part of panic disorder, but may occur in other anxiety, trauma-related, and obsessive-compulsive disorders, with substance intoxication or withdrawal, and with several medical conditions, such as hyperthyroidism. In medically healthy late adolescents and young adults, panic attacks are one of the commonest causes of episodic dizziness.

In primary anxiety disorders, dizziness and other symptoms of panic attacks are not related to vestibular dysfunction[51]; however, acute vestibular syndromes frequently cause high anxiety, including panic attacks,[52] perhaps more commonly in women than in men.[53] Regardless of gender, emergency clinicians may be confronted with patients who have coexisting medical and psychiatric causes of their episodic vestibular symptoms. Anxiety should not be overlooked in these situations because prospective studies have demonstrated that high anxiety in the midst of acute vestibular attacks is a harbinger of poor long-term outcomes. In fact, it is more predictive of chronic dizziness 3 and 12 months later than neuro-otologic variables such as the extent of peripheral vestibular loss.[54]

One of the most debilitating vestibular syndromes seen in patients who present for urgent evaluations of vestibular symptoms is PPPD, formerly known as phobic postural vertigo or chronic subjective dizziness (CSD; **Table 1**). PPPD causes chronic dizziness and unsteadiness, not acute vestibular symptoms, but it is a frequent sequela of acute vestibular syndromes such as vestibular neuritis and commonly coexists with episodic vestibular syndromes such as vestibular migraine. Triggering events for CSD include acute vestibular disorders (25%), vestibular migraine (16.5%), primary panic or generalized anxiety disorders (15% each), postconcussive syndrome (15.1%), and dysautonomia (7%).[55] Treatment of acute anxiety makes good clinical sense when patients with these problems present for emergency care, but it is not yet known if acute interventions will reduce the incidence of PPPD.

FIBROMYALGIA

A case control study of 166 fibromyalgia patients found that 63% of affected patients reported poor balance versus 4% of pain-free adults.[56] Similarly, the fibromyalgia patients from the Oslo Health Study reported symptomatic dizziness or faintness within the last week 59.3% of the time versus 26% for those without fibromyalgia.[57] An independent relationship persisted after adjustment for gender, age, comorbid conditions, and use of medications, with fibromyalgia patients having 1.92 higher odds of dizziness and faintness (95% confidence interval 1.62–2.28).

HYPERVENTILATION

Dizziness and vertigo associated with hyperventilation have a clear physiologic basis as decreased levels of blood carbon dioxide will decrease cerebral blood flow, although the mechanism may be more perceptual-cognitive.[58] Interestingly, the lightheadedness initially associated with hypocapnia can be elicited in normocarbic individuals when odors were associated with the periods of hyperventilation.[59] In general, however, hyperventilation is unlikely to be the only cause of dizziness. If causative in a patient, the sensation should be reproducible by hyperventilation and past episodes closely temporally related to hyperventilation. Consideration of the large number of medical, anxiety-related, and social factors as contributing to the initiation of and sustained nature of hyperventilation is important if this diagnosis is deemed likely.[60] **Fig. 1** provides an overview of the various diseases and social factors that may contribute to or propagate hyperventilation episodes.[61]

Table 1
Chronic subjective dizziness

Feature[a]	Description	Comments
Primary symptoms	Unsteadiness, dizziness, or both are typically present throughout the day but fluctuate in severity Symptoms are present on most days for 3 mo or more	Symptoms of CSD are usually quite persistent but wax and wane spontaneously and in response to provocative factors Vertigo is not part of CSD but CSD may coexist with other vestibular disorders. In those cases, patients may experience episodic vertigo superimposed on chronic unsteadiness and dizziness
Postural relationship	Primary symptoms are related to body posture Symptoms are most severe when walking or standing, less severe when sitting, and absent or very minor when recumbent	Some patients with CSD prefer walking to standing still, although either is more troublesome than sitting or lying down Postural and orthostatic symptoms are not the same. Postural symptoms are present while patients are in upright postures. Orthostatic symptoms occur as patients arise into an upright posture Orthostatic tremor develops while standing and improves during walking
Provocative factors (context-dependent symptom exacerbation)	Primary symptoms are present without specific provocation but are exacerbated by the following: • Active or passive motion of self that is not related to a specific direction or position • Exposure to large-field moving visual stimuli or complex (fixed or moving) visual patterns • Performance of small-field, precision visual activities (eg, reading, using a computer, fine tasks with hands)	Symptoms of CSD exist without provocation but usually reflect the cumulative burden of exposure to provocative activities throughout the day. Context-dependent factors include motion of self, exposure to environments with challenging motion stimuli, or complex visual cues and performance of visual tasks that require precise, sustained focus, such as using a computer or reading

Precipitating factors (triggering events)	Precipitating factors include: • Acute or recurrent neuro-otologic diseases that cause central or peripheral vestibular dysfunction • Acute or recurrent medical problems that produce unsteadiness or dizziness • Acute or recurrent psychiatric disorders that produce unsteadiness or dizziness	The most common triggers for CSD are: • Previous acute vestibular disorders (eg, benign paroxysmal positional vertigo, vestibular neuritis) • Episodic vestibular disorders (eg, vestibular migraine, Ménière disease) • Mild traumatic brain injury or whiplash • Panic attacks, generalized anxiety • Dysautonomias • Dysrhythmias • Adverse drug reactions and other medical events
Physical examination and laboratory findings	Physical examination and vestibular laboratory testing are often normal. Minor, nondiagnostic abnormalities occur frequently Examination and testing may reveal diagnostic evidence of a neuro-otologic or other medical condition that may be active, treated, or resolved but cannot fully explain all of the patient's symptoms	CSD may occur as an isolated condition or coexist with other neuro-otologic or medical illnesses. Positive examination findings do not necessarily exclude CSD; they may instead identify comorbid conditions At present, there are no established biomarkers for CSD, but emerging data suggest that patients may have a unique pattern of sway on static or dynamic posturography with relatively poorer performance on simpler tasks
Behavioral symptoms	Behavioral assessment may be normal. Low levels of anxiety or depression are common Behavioral assessment also may find clinically significant psychological distress, psychiatric disorders, or adverse changes in activities of daily living	Several carefully designed diagnostic studies have shown that CSD is a unique clinical entity, not a forme fruste of a psychiatric illness (see text) However, patients with CSD do have an increased prevalence of psychiatric disorders, typically anxiety or depressive disorders, compared with individuals with other neuro-otologic illnesses

[a] The first 3 features may be used to make a diagnosis of CSD. The clinical history would include 3 mo or more of persistent, posture-related unsteadiness or dizziness provoked by motion of self and one or both of the visual stimuli.

From Staab JP. Chronic subjective dizziness. Continuum (Minneap Minn) 2012;18:1121; with permission.

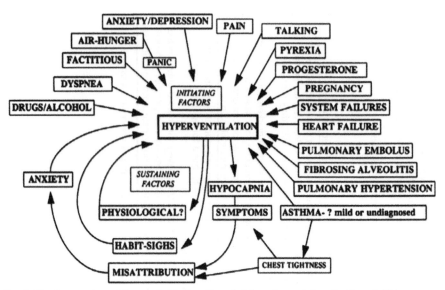

Fig. 1. The interaction of factors initiating (*top right*) and sustaining (*bottom left*) hyperventilation. A possible model for acute/subacute hyperventilation. (*From* Gardner WN. The pathophysiology of hyperventilation disorders. Chest 1996;109(2):523; with permission.)

SUMMARY

Episodic dizziness and vertigo present a diagnostic and therapeutic challenge. Although it is instructive to consider potential medical and psychiatric conditions that can induce these symptoms, it is absolutely essential to consider specific vestibular and cerebrovascular causes first. As with many serious medical conditions, substantial overlap between defined structural causes (BPPV) and other medical/psychiatric causes (orthostasis or anxiety) is likely to exist within individual patients. A rational approach to history taking, physical examination, and diagnostic testing will suggest several of these causes; a strong temporal relationship may enhance the strength of such diagnosis. In the end, dizziness is one of the most common presenting symptoms in ambulatory care, and several of the conditions described here are also extremely prevalent in the general population. As such, the consideration of medical and psychiatric causes of dizziness is important, but the consideration of these conditions should not interfere with the exclusion of defined vestibular or serious cerebrovascular causes.

REFERENCES

1. Bisdorff A, Von Brevern M, Lempert T, et al. Classification of vestibular symptoms: towards an international classification of vestibular disorders. J Vestib Res 2009; 19(1):1–13.
2. Neuhauser HK, Radtke A, von Brevern M, et al. Burden of dizziness and vertigo in the community. Arch Intern Med 2008;168(19):2118–24.
3. Bisdorff A, Bosser G, Gueguen R, et al. The epidemiology of vertigo, dizziness, and unsteadiness and its links to co-morbidities. Front Neurol 2013;4:29.
4. Bickley L, Szilagyi PG. Bates' guide to physical examination and history-taking. Riverwoods (IL): Lippincott Williams & Wilkins; 2012.

5. Newman-Toker DE. Diagnosing dizziness in the emergency department: why "what do you mean by 'dizzy'?" should not be the first question you ask [PhD]. Ann Arbor (MI): The Johns Hopkins University; 2007.

6. Carey WD. Current clinical medicine 2009: online + print. Philadelphia: Saunders/Elsevier; 2008.

7. Longo D, Fauci A, Kasper D, et al. Harrison's principles of internal medicine. New York: McGraw Hill Professional; 2011.

8. Longo DL. Harrison's online: featuring the complete contents of Harrison's principles of internal medicine. Columbus (OH): McGraw-hill; 2012.

9. Marx J, Hockberger R, Walls R. Rosen's emergency medicine—concepts and clinical practice. Oxford (United Kingdom): Elsevier Health Sciences; 2013.

10. Paulman A, Harrison JD, Nasir LS, et al. Signs and symptoms in family medicine: a literature-based approach. Oxford (United Kingdom): Elsevier Health Sciences; 2011.

11. Isaac T, Zheng J, Jha A. Use of UpToDate and outcomes in US hospitals. J Hosp Med 2012;7(2):85–90.

12. Branch W, Barton J. Approach to the patient with dizziness. Waltham (MA): UpToDate; 2014.

13. Furman J, Barton J. Evaluation of vertigo. Waltham (MA): UpToDate; 2014.

14. Newman-Toker D, Dy F, Stanton V, et al. How often is dizziness from primary cardiovascular disease true vertigo? A systematic review. J Gen Intern Med 2008; 23(12):2087–94.

15. Newman-Toker DE, Cannon LM, Stofferahn ME, et al. Imprecision in patient reports of dizziness symptom quality: a cross-sectional study conducted in an acute care setting. Mayo Clin Proc 2007;82(11):1329–40.

16. Oliver CM, Hunter SA, Ikeda T, et al. Junior doctor skill in the art of physical examination: a retrospective study of the medical admission note over four decades. BMJ Open 2013;3(4):e002257.

17. Kuruvilla A, Bhattacharya P, Rajamani K, et al. Factors associated with misdiagnosis of acute stroke in young adults. J Stroke Cerebrovasc Dis 2011;20(6):523–7.

18. Anderson JL, Adams CD, Antman EM, et al. 2011 ACCF/AHA focused update incorporated into the ACC/AHA 2007 guidelines for the management of patients with unstable angina/non-ST-elevation myocardial infarction: a report of the American College of Cardiology Foundation/American Heart Association Task Force on Practice Guidelines. Circulation 2011;123(18):e426–579.

19. Freeman R, Wieling W, Axelrod F, et al. Consensus statement on the definition of orthostatic hypotension, neurally mediated syncope and the postural tachycardia syndrome. Clin Auton Res 2011;21(2):69–72.

20. Radtke A, Lempert T, von Brevern M, et al. Prevalence and complications of orthostatic dizziness in the general population. Clin Auton Res 2011;21(3): 161–8.

21. Low PA, Opfer-Gehrking TL, McPhee BR, et al. Prospective evaluation of clinical characteristics of orthostatic hypotension. Mayo Clin Proc 1995;70(7):617–22.

22. Wu JS, Lu FH, Yang YC, et al. Postural hypotension and postural dizziness in patients with non-insulin-dependent diabetes. Arch Intern Med 1999;159(12): 1350–6.

23. Da Costa JM. On irritable heart: a clinical study of a form of functional cardiac disorder and its consequences. Am J Med 1951;11(5):559–67.

24. Peckerman A, Dahl K, Chemitiganti R, et al. Effects of posttraumatic stress disorder on cardiovascular stress responses in Gulf War veterans with fatiguing illness. Auton Neurosci 2003;108(1–2):63–72.

25. Hinton DE, Chhean D, Hofmann SG, et al. Dizziness- and palpitations-predominant orthostatic panic: physiology, flashbacks, and catastrophic cognitions. J Psychopathol Behav Assess 2008;30(2):100–10.

26. Gao Y, Lin Y, Sun K, et al. Orthostatic blood pressure dysregulation and polymorphisms of β-adrenergic receptor genes in hypertensive patients. J Clin Hypertens 2014;16(3):207–13.

27. Choi JH, Seo JD, Kim MJ, et al. Vertigo and nystagmus in orthostatic hypotension. Eur J Neurol 2015;22(4):648–55.

28. Low PA, Sandroni P, Joyner M, et al. Postural tachycardia syndrome (POTS). J Cardiovasc Electrophysiol 2009;20(3):352–8.

29. Thieben MJ, Sandroni P, Sletten DM, et al. Postural orthostatic tachycardia syndrome: the Mayo Clinic experience. Mayo Clin Proc 2007;82(3):308–13.

30. Benarroch EE. Postural tachycardia syndrome: a heterogeneous and multifactorial disorder. Mayo Clin Proc 2012;87(12):1214–25.

31. Benrud-Larson LM, Sandroni P, Haythornthwaite JA, et al. Correlates of functional disability in patients with postural tachycardia syndrome: preliminary cross-sectional findings. Health Psychol 2003;22(6):643–8.

32. Parsaik A, Allison TG, Singer W, et al. Deconditioning in patients with orthostatic intolerance. Neurology 2012;79(14):1435–9.

33. Moya A, Sutton R, Ammirati F, et al. Guidelines for the diagnosis and management of syncope (version 2009). Eur Heart J 2009;30:2631–71.

34. Thiruganasambandamoorthy V, Stiell IG, Wells GA, et al. Outcomes in presyncope patients: a prospective cohort study. Ann Emerg Med 2015;65(3):268–76.e266.

35. Muppa P, Sheldon RS, McRae M, et al. Gynecological and menstrual disorders in women with vasovagal syncope. Clin Auton Res 2013;23(3):117–22.

36. Ullman E, Edlow JA. Complete heart block complicating the head impulse test. Arch Neurol 2010;67(10):1272–4.

37. Goto F, Tsutsumi T, Nakamura I, et al. Neurally mediated syncope presenting with paroxysmal positional vertigo and tinnitus. Auris Nasus Larynx 2012;39(5):531–3.

38. Staab JP, Ruckenstein MJ. Autonomic nervous system function in chronic dizziness. Otol Neurotol 2007;28(6):854–9.

39. Chimirri S, Aiello R, Mazzitello C, et al. Vertigo/dizziness as a drugs' adverse reaction. J Pharmacol Pharmacother 2013;4(Suppl 1):S104–9.

40. Haddad PM. Antidepressant discontinuation syndromes. Drug Saf 2001;24(3):183–97.

41. Timbo BB, Ross MP, McCarthy PV, et al. Dietary supplements in a national survey: prevalence of use and reports of adverse events. J Am Diet Assoc 2006;106(12):1966–74.

42. Mangabeira Albernaz PL, Fukuda Y. Glucose, insulin and inner ear pathology. Acta Otolaryngol 1984;97(5–6):496–501.

43. Rybak LP. Metabolic disorders of the vestibular system. Otolaryngol Head Neck Surg 1995;112(1):128–32.

44. Penney DG. Carbon monoxide poisoning. Boca Raton (FL): Taylor & Francis; 2007.

45. Weaver LK. Carbon monoxide poisoning. N Engl J Med 2009;360(12):1217–25.

46. Bronstein AM. Vision and vertigo: some visual aspects of vestibular disorders. J Neurol 2004;251(4):381–7.

47. Balaban CD, Jacob RG. Background and history of the interface between anxiety and vertigo. J Anxiety Disord 2001;15(1–2):27–51.

48. Bayrak IK, Durmus D, Bayrak AO, et al. Effect of cervical spondylosis on vertebral arterial flow and its association with vertigo. Clin Rheumatol 2009;28(1):59–64.
49. Machaly SA, Senna MK, Sadek AG. Vertigo is associated with advanced degenerative changes in patients with cervical spondylosis. Clin Rheumatol 2011; 30(12):1527–34.
50. DSM-5 Diagnostic classification. Diagnostic and statistical manual of mental disorders. 2013.
51. Furman JM, Jacob RG. Psychiatric dizziness. Neurology 1997;48(5):1161–6.
52. Pollak L, Klein C, Rafael S, et al. Anxiety in the first attack of vertigo. Otolaryngol Head Neck Surg 2003;128(6):829–34.
53. Ferrari S, Monzani D, Baraldi S, et al. Vertigo "in the pink": the impact of female gender on psychiatric-psychosomatic comorbidity in benign paroxysmal positional vertigo patients. Psychosomatics 2014;55(3):280–8.
54. Godemann F, Siefert K, Hantschke-Brüggemann M, et al. What accounts for vertigo one year after neuritis vestibularis – anxiety or a dysfunctional vestibular organ? J Psychiatr Res 2005;39(5):529–34.
55. Staab JP, Ruckenstein MJ. Expanding the differential diagnosis of chronic dizziness. Arch Otolaryngol Head Neck Surg 2007;133(2):170–6.
56. Watson NF, Buchwald D, Goldberg J, et al. Neurologic signs and symptoms in fibromyalgia. Arthritis Rheum 2009;60(9):2839–44.
57. Tamber AL, Bruusgaard D. Self-reported faintness or dizziness – comorbidity and use of medicines. An epidemiological study. Scand J Public Health 2009;37(6): 613–20.
58. Bresseleers J, Van Diest I, De Peuter S, et al. Feeling lightheaded: the role of cerebral blood flow. Psychosom Med 2010;72(7):672–80.
59. Van Diest I, De Peuter S, Piedfort K, et al. Acquired lightheadedness in response to odors after hyperventilation. Psychosom Med 2006;68(2):340–7.
60. Brashear R. Hyperventilation syndrome. Lung 1983;161(1):257–73.
61. Gardner WN. The pathophysiology of hyperventilation disorders. Chest 1996; 109(2):516–34.

Section III – Acute, Continuous Dizziness and Vertigo

Early Diagnosis and Treatment of Traumatic Vestibulopathy and Postconcussive Dizziness

Michael E. Hoffer, MD[a],*, Michael C. Schubert, PT, PhD[b,c],
Carey D. Balaban, PhD[d,e,f,g]

KEYWORDS

- Mild traumatic brain injury (mTBI) • Neurosensory sequelae • Dizziness
- Vestibular rehabilitation

KEY POINTS

- Neurosensory disorders are the most common sequelae of mild traumatic brain injury (mTBI), and among these, balance disorders are the ones most frequently seen.
- Balance disorders seen after mTBI can be diagnosed and treated, and whereas some resolve with time, many of these disorders require treatment.
- Vestibular rehabilitation is one of the most important treatment modalities available for patients with mTBI and has been documented to be successful in this patient group.
- Untreated mTBI can produce long-term degenerative neurosensory disorders.

INTRODUCTION

mTBI is an increasingly common public health concern that has garnered increased attention in both the lay press and medical literature. Neurosensory effects are among the most common sequelae of mTBI, with balance-related findings being the most

[a] Department of Otolaryngology, University of Miami, 1120 Northwest 14th Street, CRB 5th Floor, Miami, FL 33136, USA; [b] Department of Otolaryngology Head and Neck Surgery, The Johns Hopkins University School of Medicine, 601 North Caroline Street, Room 6245, Baltimore, MD 21287, USA; [c] Department of Physical Medicine and Rehabilitation, The Johns Hopkins University School of Medicine, 601 North Caroline Street, Room 6245, Baltimore, MD 21287, USA; [d] Department of Otolaryngology, Eye and Ear Institute, University of Pittsburgh, Suite 107, 200 Lothrop Street, Pittsburgh, PA 15213, USA; [e] Department of Neurobiology, Eye and Ear Institute, University of Pittsburgh, Suite 107, 200 Lothrop Street, Pittsburgh, PA 15213, USA; [f] Department of Communication Science & Disorders, University of Pittsburgh, Suite 107, 200 Lothrop Street, Pittsburgh, PA 15213, USA; [g] Department of Bioengineering, Eye and Ear Institute, University of Pittsburgh, Suite 107, 200 Lothrop Street, Pittsburgh, PA 15213, USA
* Corresponding author.
E-mail address: Michael.hoffer@miami.edu

Neurol Clin 33 (2015) 661–668
http://dx.doi.org/10.1016/j.ncl.2015.04.004
0733-8619/15/$ – see front matter © 2015 Elsevier Inc. All rights reserved.
neurologic.theclinics.com

common.[1–6] Balance disorders present a unique opportunity with respect to mTBI because they are almost universally present, they can be documented easily with qualitative and quantitative tests, and prompt treatment can result in marked improvement and return to function. On the other hand, untreated acute balance disorders after mTBI represent a significant and underappreciated public health issue. Chronic balance issues from mTBI can affect quality of life for many years after the injury and, in some cases, balance function can deteriorate unpredictably over time. The vestibular system itself has been shown to be damaged in mTBI as evidenced by documented benign paroxysmal positional vertigo caused by blast or blunt trauma mechanisms,[7] semicircular canal dehiscence,[8] and peripheral vestibular hypofunction.[8] This article begins with a review of the prevalence of mTBI in general, and then discusses clinical evidence indicating balance disorders after mTBI and examines the most recent trends in diagnosis. Finally, it discusses the recent basic scientific hypotheses regarding the cause of mTBI-induced neurosensory disorders and provides a brief overview of vestibular rehabilitation for mTBI.

THE DEFINITION OF MILD TRAUMATIC BRAIN INJURY

There are a variety of definitions of mTBI. Although these definitions were developed by health organizations and government agencies, there is no consensus definition. For a detailed discussion of this particular topic, the reader is referred to the Centers for Disease Control and Prevention (CDC) Web site,[5] which is an excellent resource for traumatic brain injury (TBI)- and mTBI-related health issues. For this article, the authors have adopted a basic functional definition of TBI as follows:

1. A traumatic event affecting the head (such as blunt trauma, explosion, or large acceleration-deceleration)
2. An event that resulted in alteration or loss of consciousness
3. An event with resultant neurologic symptoms and signs

Among individuals with such events, mTBI is defined by the following inclusion criteria:

1. Glasgow Coma Score greater than 13
2. Loss of consciousness for less than 1 hour
3. No surgical intervention needed (including a burr hole for drainage of bleeding)

Stated simply, mTBI (as the authors address it in this article) is a concussion. Although penetrating injuries can cause TBI, they are rarely mild and are generally associated with other types of disorders, so penetrating TBI is not addressed in this article.

EPIDEMIOLOGY

It is difficult to draw reliable conclusions from the existing epidemiologic data regarding prevalence and long-term consequences of mTBI. The lack of consensus in definitions and the fact that many mTBI cases go unreported makes epidemiologic classification problematic. It is clear that the reported prevalence of mTBI is increasing. Several reports focused on selected populations, such as high-school athletes[9] or emergency departments (EDs), over limited time frames[10,11] do give estimates of the relative prevalence of mTBI in different populations. A recent study by Marin and colleagues[12] used the Nationwide Emergency Department Sample to investigate trends of visits to ED for TBI between 2006 and 2010. The data culled from a sample of 950 hospitals showed a sharp increase in the weighted rates of

ED visits from 2006 to 2010. There were 637 TBI visits per 100,000 ED visits in 2006, and by 2010, this figure was up to 822 per 100,000, with a disproportionate increase in the number of reported mTBI or concussion visits.[11] What also seems to be apparent is that mTBI occurs preferentially in certain age groups. The CDC reported that almost 75% of all TBI visits were from individuals aged 0 to 4 years or older than 65 years.[1] This 75% figure is likely an overestimate because of underreporting from the 5- to 64-year-old segment of the population.

Certain established trends in TBI include a preponderance in men older than 75 years and motor vehicle accidents being the most common cause of TBI in individuals aged 15 to 24 years.[13] It is hard to know if these observations apply to mTBI as well. Although football injuries receive the most attention in the press,[14] there is a substantial literature regarding the occupational incidence of mTBI from the military alone.[1–5,15–17]

BALANCE DISORDERS AFTER BLAST INJURIES

There have been several studies examining balance disorders after blast exposure. An explosives detonation produces a shock wave, a blast wind, and an electromagnetic pulse. Primary blast injury is produced by shock wave propagation through tissue. The leading edge of the shock wave, the blast front, is an overpressure that propagates supersonically; it is followed by a negative pressure termed the underpressure. Reflections off environmental surfaces can produce more complicated exposures and greater injury. A single overpressure-underpressure blast wave sequence, described by a Friedlander wave profile, propagates into the brain case as a positive-negative shift in intracranial pressure.[18,19] Computer simulation studies have estimated deformations of the brain from blast waves,[20] which predict the greatest peak-to-peak effects in the posterior fossa.[21] Secondary blast injury is produced by shrapnel or fragments. Tertiary blast injury can produce blunt trauma by impact with objects in the environment. Quaternary blast injury is produced by other detonation products such as heat, electromagnetic pulses, and detonation toxins.

Hoffer and colleagues[1] described the symptom complex in blast-exposed service members with primary blast mTBI in the acute (81 subjects, within 72 hours), subacute (25 subjects, 4–30 days), and chronic (42 subjects, >30 days) periods.[1] Significant differences were noted in the prevalence of dizziness among the acute group (98%) compared with the subacute (76%) and chronic (84%) groups. Also, there was a significant difference in vertigo prevalence: 4% in the acute group, in contrast to 47% and 36% in the subacute and chronic groups, respectively. There was no statistical difference in frequency of hearing loss (33%–49%) and headache (72%–82%). From these data, 4 descriptive diagnostic classifications were established for dizziness after blast exposure: positional vertigo, post-blast-induced dizziness, postblast exercise-induced dizziness, and blast-induced dizziness with vertigo. These categories help to differentiate these patients from the more well-known entity of blunt trauma TBI (concussion). Differences include more constant symptom presence and dizziness that occurs during exertion rather than after exertion. Eye movements during rotational chair testing suggested worsening horizontal vestibuloocular reflex (VOR) function over time, but a larger study is needed to draw statistically sound conclusions.

Scherer and colleagues[2] examined vestibular test results in a group of blast-exposed service members divided into 2 groups based on the presence or absence of vestibular symptoms. In both groups, 83% had a concomitant blast and blunt trauma. All subjects were examined at least 30 days postinjury except for 1 symptomatic subject examined 14 days from injury. Each group had 12 subjects.

Videonystagmography results were abnormal in both groups, although slightly (but not significantly) more prevalent in the symptomatic group (6/12 vs 4/12). The rotational chair testing showed more of a difference between the 2 groups with 6 of 12 symptomatic patients exhibiting abnormalities in contrast to 1 of 10 in the asymptomatic group. Again, small sample size precluded any definitive conclusions. The abnormal videonystagmography results in the nonsymptomatic side were thought to be due to confounding medications and possible central pathology. Subjective self-report measures were significantly different between the 2 groups. The same group of patients was examined by Scherer and colleagues[22] who reported their results separately. This study was statistically powered to 0.80 with 12 subjects each, and active and passive head impulse testing was performed resulting in 4 different impulse rotation conditions: passive yaw, active yaw, passive pitch, and active pitch. Only 11 subjects from each group were reported because of excessive noise during signal recording for 2 subjects. Gain differences were found for active yaw and active and passive pitch, although there was variability in the findings. For example, 6 of 12 symptomatic subjects displayed angular VOR gains less than 0.85 indicating vestibular hypofunction, yet 2 of 12 had abnormally elevated gains that indicated cerebellar pathology. The study also included correlation of the angular VOR with vestibular symptoms during exertion. Passive pitch angular VOR gain showed an association, although the study was not adequately powered to draw definitive conclusions. Nonetheless, it suggests a possible avenue of investigation to find an objective measure of postblast exercise-induced dizziness that may be used as an outcome measure to establish fitness for duty.

Finally, Akin and Murnane[23] published an overview of blast injury and chronic vestibular consequences. In addition to their summary of findings over the past several years, they also published preliminary data for 31 symptomatic patients with long-term blast mTBI and/or blunt-impact induced mTBI seen in the Mountain Home Veterans Affairs Medical Center Vestibular/Balance Laboratory. Otolith dysfunction, manifested by abnormal cervical vestibular evoked myogenic potentials and/or abnormal judgments of subjective visual vertical in static and/or dynamic conditions, was present in 26 of 31 (84%) patients. In addition, 29% had caloric weakness and/or abnormal rotational chair results. The long-term prominence of these signs is consistent with our earlier report[1] of increasingly severe impairment when the first presentation is more than 30 days after injury.

BALANCE DISORDERS AFTER BLUNT HEAD INJURY

Blunt head injury has a well-known association with balance disorders.[24–26] Suarez and colleagues[24] demonstrated that the dizziness was one of the most frequent symptoms seen after mild head injury in a civilian setting. Meanwhile, Grubenhoff[25] examined the relative frequency of specific types of dizziness as a function of age in an mTBI group and found that younger individuals were more susceptible to potentially treatable causes of balance disorders. Hoffer and colleagues[27] examined blunt head trauma in a military population and characterized the dizziness seen after this type of trauma as a common symptom with patterns of dizziness different from the pattern that occurs after primary blast injury.

DIAGNOSIS

Diagnosis of mTBI has always presented challenges. This fact is true in part because many of the symptoms are self-reported with variable intensity over time. As discussed earlier, balance disorders present a unique window into the brain for diagnosing mTBI. One of the most interesting and promising areas includes examining optokinetic and vestibular reflexes in response to a variety of visual and vestibular challenges. Working with Neuro Kinetics, Inc (Pittsburgh, PA, USA), the authors have described that a combination of oculomotor, vestibular, and symptom measures can discriminate patients with mTBI from control subjects.[28–30] Patients with acute mTBI can be identified with greater than 90% selectivity and sensitivity with a test battery that includes saccade testing (saccades, antisaccades, and saccadic reaction times), smooth pursuit performance, vestibular performance (harmonic rotation, visual enhancement/suppression of the horizontal, and head impulse testing), optokinetic testing, as well as self-reports of posttraumatic migrainelike symptoms. Other groups have similarly reported consistent eye movement findings. In 60 individuals with chronic mTBI, oculomotor testing revealed position and velocity error as well as saccadic intrusions, as measured using a head-mounted tracker attached to binocular cameras to track eye movement in response to visual or motion stimuli.[31]

Although not specific to balance disorders, other recent and relevant work investigating mTBI diagnosis is enlightening. A study in vision performed by the Veterans Administration led to the development of a 17-item tool designed to work in concert with 7 specific eye tests.[32] Magnetoencephalography was used to examine a large series of patients with mTBI and reported a specificity of 87% for correctly identifying mTBI.[33] Emergency and point-of-service diagnostic techniques for mTBI include the King-Devick test, sports concussion assessment tool (SCAT-2) test, acute concussion evaluation tool, and immediate post- concussion assessment and cognitive testing (ImPACT) test.[34–37] Although none of these tests focus exclusively on balance, each of them relies on balance elements in the test. For an extended review of imaging technologies, beyond the scope of this article, the reader is referred to an excellent article that summarizes functional MRI findings.[33]

TREATMENT

Advances in treatment of mTBI have been relatively slow to develop. In general, treatment can be classified as pharmacotherapy and rehabilitation. To date, the only pharmacotherapy that has demonstrated effectiveness is N-acetyl cysteine (NAC). NAC was found to be an effective countermeasure for blast-induced mTBI.[38] Working in a combat environment, a double-blinded placebo-controlled study revealed that NAC was far more effective than a control medicine at reducing symptoms measured at 7 days postinjury. Other pharmacologic methods are in development, but none have gone to clinical studies as yet. Work must be continued in this area. At present, therefore, the mainstay of treatment remains physical therapy.

The type of physical therapy that has been shown to be most effective and most common in treating patients with mTBI is vestibular rehabilitation.[39] Vestibular physical therapy (VPT) is a subspecialization within physical therapy that requires patients with dizziness and balance disorders to perform challenging postural, gait, and gaze stability tasks. Most VPT programs prescribe exercises to be done multiple times at home, presuming the patient is compliant and can do the exercises safely. The VPT may also involve outpatient visits. While there exists a significant body of literature examining the benefit of VPT in vestibular pathology,[40] there is an ever-increasing amount of evidence to support its role in treating mTBI. Alsalaheen and colleagues[41] have shown that vestibular rehabilitation improves outcomes and shortens disability times in patients with mTBI that did not improve with rest alone. Gottshall has demonstrated that return to work rates in this population is dramatically improved by vestibular rehabilitation. In order to study recovery more closely, Gottshall[42] developed a battery of vestibular-visual-cognitive tests for establishing initial vestibular function and tracking the effectiveness of the VPT. The battery included the sensory organization test and motor control test as part of computerized dynamic posturography, static visual acuity, perception time, target acquisition, target following, dynamic visual acuity, and gaze stabilization tests (as part of the vestibular-visual-cognitive function testing with the Neurocom inVision Tunnel [Nuerocom Inc, Clakmas, OR, USA]). Performance was assessed at 0, 4, and 8 weeks from injury. The results were compared with previously collected, unpublished normative data. After 8 weeks, target following and dynamic visual acuity normalized. Although gaze stabilization scores improved, they did not approach normative levels within the 8-week time frame.[42]

Others have focused on different types of therapy, which have also been shown to be productive. Many individuals will have difficulty when attempting to read near targets because of the required convergence of the eyes creating symptoms or difficulty to physically perform. Thiagarajan and colleagues[43] trained subjects to do ocular fixation, predictable saccades, and simulated reading exercises in patients with vergence deficiency. The investigators not only found improvement in symptoms but also found significant improvement in errors in horizontal vergence.[43] Cervical spine physical therapy was shown to resolve symptoms in 73% of 15 patients with mTBI compared with only 7% in a control group.[44]

SUMMARY

mTBI is an increasingly common public health issue. Most of the acute, subacute, and chronic symptoms are neurosensory in nature and most commonly cause dizziness. Recognizing dizziness in this population is important because it provides a starting point for management of a difficult clinical entity, which can be measured objectively and treated effectively. Vestibular rehabilitation remains the standard treatment of mTBI, although clinical trials in the effectiveness of both rehabilitation and pharmacologic management are lacking.

REFERENCES

1. Hoffer ME, Balaban C, Gottshall K, et al. Blast exposure: vestibular consequences and associated characteristics. Otol Neurotol 2010;31(2):232–6.
2. Scherer MR, Burrows H, Pinto R, et al. Evidence of central and peripheral vestibular pathology in blast-related traumatic brain injury. Otol Neurotol 2011;32(4): 571–80.
3. Hoge CW, McGurk D, Thomas JL, et al. Mild traumatic brain injury in U.S. Soldiers returning from Iraq. N Engl J Med 2008;358:453–63.
4. Terrio H, Brenner LA, Ivins BJ, et al. Traumatic brain injury screening: preliminary findings in a US Army Brigade Combat Team. J Head Trauma Rehabil 2009;24: 14–23.
5. Available at: http://www.cdc.gov/TraumaticBrainInjury/index.html. Accessed March 27, 2015.
6. Hosek B. How is deployment to Iraq and Afghanistan affecting U.S. service members and their families? An overview of early RAND research on the topic. Santa Monica (CA): RAND Corporation; 2011.
7. Pisani V1, Mazzone S, Di Mauro R, et al. A survey of the nature of trauma of post-traumatic benign paroxysmal positional vertigo. Int J Audiol 2015;54(5):329–33.
8. Honaker JA1, Lester HF, Patterson JN, et al. Examining postconcussion symptoms of dizziness and imbalance on neurocognitive performance in collegiate football players. Otol Neurotol 2014;35(6):1111–7.

9. Powell JW, Barber-Foss KD. Traumatic Brain Injury in High School Athlete. JAMA 1999;282(10):958–63.
10. Guerrero JL, Thurman DJ, Sniezek JE. Emergency department visits associated with traumatic brain injury: United States, 1995-1996. Brain Inj 2000; 14(2):181–6.
11. Kerr ZY, Harmon KJ, Marshall SW, et al. The epidemiology of traumatic brain injuries treated in emergency departments in North Carolina, 2010–2011. N C Med J 2014;75(1):8–14.
12. Marin JR, Weaver MD, Yealy DM, et al. Trends in visits for traumatic brain injury to emergency departments in the United States. JAMA 2014;311(18):1917–9.
13. Lagbas C, Bazargan-Hejazi S, Shaheen M, et al. Traumatic brain injury related hospitalization and mortality in California. Biomed Res Int 2013;2013:143092.
14. Olson D, Sikka RS, Labounty A, et al. Injuries in professional football: current concepts. Curr Sports Med Rep 2013;12(6):381–90.
15. Shah A, Ayala M, Capra G, et al. Otologic assessment of blast and nonblast injury in returning middle east-deployed service members. Laryngoscope 2014;124(1): 272–7.
16. Johnson CM, Perez CF, Hoffer ME. The implications of physical injury on otovestibular and cognitive symptomatology following blast exposure. Otolaryngol Head Neck Surg 2014;150(3):437–40.
17. Bryan CJ. Multiple traumatic brain injury and concussive symptoms among deployed military personnel. Brain Inj 2013;27(12):1333–7.
18. Stuhmiller JH, Phillips YY, Richmond DR. The physics and mechanisms of primary blast injury. In: Bellamy RF, Zajtchuk R, editors. Textbook of military medicine. conventional warfare: blast, ballistic and burn injuries. Washington, DC: Department of the Army, Office of the Surgeon General, Borden Institute; 1990. p. 241–70.
19. Chavko M, Koller WA, Prusaczyk WK, et al. Measurement of blast wave by a miniature fiber optic pressure transducer in the rat brain. J Neurosci Methods 2007; 159:277–81.
20. Moore DF, Jerusalem A, Nyein M, et al. Computational biology–modeling of primary blast effects on the central nervous system. Neuroimage 2009;47:T10–20.
21. Wang C, Pahk JB, Balaban CD, et al. Computational study of human head response to primary blast waves of five levels from three directions. PLoS One 2014;9(11):e113264.
22. Scherer MR, Shelhamer MJ, Schubert MC. Characterizing high-velocity angular vestibule-ocular reflex function in service member's post-blast exposure. Exp Brain Res 2011;208:399–410.
23. Akin FW, Murnane OD. Head injury and blast exposure: vestibular consequences. Otolaryngol Clin North Am 2011;44(2):323–34.
24. Suarez H, Alonso R, Arocena M, et al. Clinical characteristics of positional vertigo after mild head trauma. Acta Otolaryngol 2011;131(4):377–81.
25. Grubenhoff JA, Kirkwood MW, Deakyne S, et al. Detailed concussion symptom analysis in a paediatric ED population. Brain Inj 2011;25(10):943–9.
26. Gottshall K, Drake A, Gray N, et al. Objective vestibular tests as outcome measures in head injury patients. Laryngoscope 2003;113(10):1746–50.
27. Hoffer ME, Donaldson C, Gottshall KR, et al. Blunt and blast head trauma: different entities. Int Tinnitus J 2009;15(2):115–8.
28. Hoffer ME, Braverman A, Crawford J, et al. Assessment of oculomotor, vestibular and reaction time response following a concussive event. Presented at the 2015 Midwinter Meeting of the Association for Research in Otolaryngology. Baltimore, MD, February 21–25, 2015.

29. Balaban CD, Braverman A, Crawford J, et al. Optokinetic Fast phase and saccade motor performance are depressed in acute concussion/mild traumatic brain injury. Presented at the 2015 Midwinter Meeting of the Association for Research in Otolaryngology. Baltimore, MD, February 21–25, 2015.

30. Kiderman A, Hoffer ME, Braverman A, et al. Comparing oculomotor and optokinetic findings to symptoms in patients with acute mTBI. Presented at the 2015 Midwinter Meeting of the Association for Research in Otolaryngology. Baltimore, MD, February 21–25, 2015.

31. Cifu DX, Wares JR, Hoke KW, et al. Differential eye movements in mild traumatic brain injury versus normal controls. J Head Trauma Rehabil 2015;30(1):21–8. Superb analysis of eye movement issues from specialized VA group focusing on TBI.

32. Goodrich GL, Martinsen GL, Flyg HM, et al. U.S. Department of Veterans Affairs. Development of a mild traumatic brain injury-specific vision screening protocol: a Delphi study. J Rehabil Res Dev 2013;50(6):757–68.

33. Lee RR, Huang M. Magnetoencephalography in the diagnosis of concussion. Prog Neurol Surg 2014;28:94–111 (Excellent review of MEG).

34. Eierud C, Craddock RC, Fletcher S, et al. Neuroimage Clin 2014;4:283–94.

35. Silverberg ND, Luoto TM, Ohman J, et al. Assessment of mild traumatic brain injury with the King-Devick Test in an emergency department sample. Brain Inj 2014;28:1–4.

36. Zuckerbraun NS, Atabaki S, Collins MW, et al. Use of modified acute concussion evaluation tools in the emergency department. Pediatrics 2014;133(4):635–42.

37. Gómez PA, de-la-Cruz J, Lora D, et al. Validation of a prognostic score for early mortality in severe head injury cases. J Neurosurg 2014;121(6):1314–22.

38. Hoffer ME, Balaban C, Slade MD, et al. Amelioration of acute sequelae of blast induced mild traumatic brain injury by N-acetyl cysteine: a double-blind, Placebo Controlled Study. PLoS One 2013;8(1):e54163.

39. Alsalaheen BA, Whitney SL, Mucha A, et al. Exercise prescription patterns in patients treated with vestibular rehabilitation after concussion. Physiother Res Int 2013;18(2):100–8.

40. McDonnell MN, Hillier SL. Vestibular rehabilitation for unilateral peripheral vestibular dysfunction. Cochrane Database Syst Rev 2015;(1):CD005397.

41. Alsalaheen BA, Mucha A, Morris LO, et al. Vestibular rehabilitation for dizziness and balance disorders after concussion. J Neurol Phys Ther 2010;34(2):87–93.

42. Gottshall KR, Hoffer ME. Tracking recovery of vestibular function in individuals with blast-induced head trauma using vestibular-visual-cognitive interaction tests. J Neurol Phys Ther 2010;34(2):94–7.

43. Thiagarajan P, Ciuffreda KJ. Versional eye tracking in mild traumatic brain injury (mTBI): effects of oculomotor training (OMT). Brain Inj 2014;28(7):930–43.

44. Schneider KJ, Meeuwisse WH, Nettel-Aguirre A, et al. Cervicovestibular rehabilitation in sport-related concussion: a randomized controlled trial. Br J Sports Med 2014;48(17):1294–8.

Acute Unilateral Vestibulopathy

Michael Strupp, MD, FANA, FEAN[a],*, Mans Magnusson, MD[b]

KEYWORDS

- Vertigo • Vestibular neuritis • Nystagmus • Vestibulopathy

KEY POINTS

- Normal vestibular end organs generate an equal resting-firing frequency of the axons, which is the same on both sides under static conditions. An acute unilateral vestibulopathy leads to a vestibular tone imbalance.
- Acute unilateral vestibulopathy is defined by the patient history and the clinical examination and, in unclear cases, laboratory examinations. Key signs and symptoms are an acute onset of spinning vertigo, postural imbalance and nausea as well as a horizontal rotatory nystagmus beating towards the non-affected side, a pathological head-impulse test and no evidence for central vestibular or ocular motor dysfunction. The so-called big five allow a differentiation between a peripheral and central lesion by the bedside examination.
- The differential diagnosis of peripheral labyrinthine and vestibular nerve disorders mimicking acute unilateral vestibulopathy includes central vestibular disorders, in particular "vestibular pseudoneuritis" and other peripheral vestibular disorders, such as beginning Menière's disease.
- The management of acute unilateral vestibulopathy involves (1) symptomatic treatment with antivertiginous drugs, (2) causal treatment with corticosteroids, and (3) physical therapy.

 Videos of spontaneous horizontal nystagmus to the right with a very low intensity during fixation; blocking visual fixation with M glasses; head-impulse testing; pathological Romberg testing with a fall to the left after closing the eyes; and pathological tandem Romberg with a fall to the left after closing the eyes accompany this article at http://www.neurologic.theclinics.com/

CASE SCENARIO

A 56-year-old male reported that he had been suffering from acute onset of spinning vertigo, unsteadiness with a tendency to fall to the left and nausea for one day. When

---

[a] Department of Neurology, German Center for Vertigo and Balance Disorders, University Hospital Munich, Campus Grosshadern, Munich 81377, Germany; [b] Department of Otolaryngology, Lund University, Lund 22100, Sweden
* Corresponding author.
E-mail address: michael.strupp@med.uni-muenchen.de

Neurol Clin 33 (2015) 669–685
http://dx.doi.org/10.1016/j.ncl.2015.04.012   **neurologic.theclinics.com**
0733-8619/15/$ – see front matter © 2015 Elsevier Inc. All rights reserved.

he tried to fixate anything, the image of the visual surroundings moved. He had no history of prior attacks or episodes of vertigo or dizziness. He did not suffer from decreased hearing, ringing in the ears, headache, or hypersensitivity to light or sound.

The clinical examination revealed a spontaneous horizontal nystagmus to the right with a very low intensity during fixation (Video 1). Its intensity increased during convergence and when looking to the right. When blocking visual fixation with Frenzel's or M glasses the intensity of the nystagmus significantly increased (Video 2) which is typical of a peripheral vestibular spontaneous nystagmus. The head-impulse test was pathological on the left (Video 3). There was no skew-deviation/vertical misalignment and no evidence for direction-changing, gaze-evoked nystagmus. Hearing was normal. Romberg testing (Video 4) and tandem Romberg (Video 5) revealed a tendency to fall to the left. The video-head impulse test showed a horizontal angular vestibulo-ocular reflex (VOR) gain of 0.4 on the right and of 0.85 on the left. Caloric testing revealed a significant hypo-responsiveness on the right. Cervical vestibular-evoked myogenic potentials (cVEMPs) were normal on both sides. The amplitudes of the ocular vestibular-evoked myogenic potentials (oVEMPs) were reduced on the right. Based on the patient history, the bedside examination, and the laboratory examinations, the diagnosis of acute unilateral vestibulopathy was made. The patient was treated with 100 mg per day methylprednisolone; the dosage was tapered every fourth day by 20 mg. From day three the patient also performed vestibular exercises and balance training three times per day. He recovered gradually over several weeks.

PREVALENCE AND PATHOMECHANISMS
Epidemiology

Based on current criteria for state-of-the-art epidemiologic studies, there are no valid data on the prevalence of acute unilateral vestibulopathy.[1] An annual incidence of between 3.5 and 15.5 per 100,000 persons has been described.[2,3] In a large cohort of more than 22,000 patients who had standardized evaluations in a vertigo clinic, acute unilateral vestibulopathy was the sixth most common cause of vertigo/dizziness and the third most common cause of peripheral vestibular disorders (benign paroxysmal positional vertigo [BPPV] ranks first, Menière's disease second). It accounts for about 8% of patients with vertigo[4]; this is also true for children.[5] The usual age of onset is between 30 and 60 years,[3] and age distribution plateaus between 40 and 50 years.[2,3] There is no significant gender difference. The reported recurrence rate varies between 1.9%[6] and 10.7%.[7]

Etiology

The most popular theory is that of a viral cause, but the evidence for it remains circumstantial (see Refs.[8,9]). The following arguments are presented to support a viral cause.[1] Vestibular nerve histopathology in cases of acute unilateral vestibulopathy is similar to that seen in single cases of herpes zoster oticus, when temporal bone histopathology was available.[2] An animal model of vestibular nuclei (VN) was developed by inoculating herpes simplex virus (HSV)-1 into the auricle of mice.[3] HSV-1 DNA was repeatedly detected in about two-thirds of autopsied human vestibular ganglia by polymerase chain reaction[10]; further the latency-associated transcript was found in about 70% of human vestibular ganglia.[11] All these findings indicate that the vestibular ganglia, like other cranial nerve ganglia, are latently infected by HSV-1. A similar cause is also assumed for Bell palsy and supported by the demonstration of HSV-1 DNA in the endoneurial fluid of affected subjects. If HSV is the most likely candidate, it can be assumed to reside in a latent state in the vestibular ganglia, for example, in the ganglionic nuclei as reported in other cranial nerves. As a result of intercurrent factors, it is thought that the virus suddenly replicates, inducing inflammation and edema, causing secondary cell damage of the vestibular ganglion cells and axons in the bony channels of the skull through which the vestibular nerve passes. Because the channel housing the superior vestibular nerve is 7 times longer and has more speculae[12] and the posterior semicircular canal is innervated by an additional anastomosis,[13] this may explain why the posterior semicircular canal is often but not always spared (see Pathophysiology). Despite these findings, a viral cause has not yet been conclusively proven. The lack of compelling structural evidence for even a consistent inflammatory component has raised doubt about terms that imply an inflammatory pathomechanism, such as vestibular neuritis or labyrinthitis, leading to a preference for acute unilateral vestibulopathy.

Pathophysiology

Peripheral vestibular spontaneous nystagmus
Normal vestibular end organs generate an equal resting-firing frequency of the axons, which is the same on both sides. This continuous excitation (resting discharge rate in monkey ≈ 100 Hz; 1800 vestibular afferents for each labyrinth, ie, 1.8 million action potentials per second) is transmitted to the VN via vestibular nerves. Pathologic processes affecting an end organ or vestibular nerve alter its firing frequency (generally a reduction in firing), thereby creating a vestibular tone imbalance. This imbalance causes spontaneous nystagmus with the slow phase (which is the pathologic component of the nystagmus) of the eye movements toward the impaired labyrinth. This imbalance is also the cause of the other manifestations on different levels, that is, perceptual (rotatory vertigo, displacement of the subjective vertical), ocular motor (ocular torsion in addition to spontaneous nystagmus), postural, and vegetative (nausea).

Lesion location
The 3-dimensional features of the spontaneous nystagmus, that is, the horizontal, vertical, and torsional components and the dynamic deficit of the VOR of the horizontal, anterior, and posterior semicircular canals were measured in acute unilateral vestibulopathy by means of the scleral coil technique and analyzed by a vector analysis in 1996.[14] These measurements supported the earlier view[15] that acute unilateral vestibulopathy is, in most cases, a partial rather than a total unilateral vestibular lesion. Specifically, it often affects the superior division of the vestibular nerve (innervating the horizontal and anterior semicircular canals, the maculae of the utricle, and the anterosuperior part of the sacculus), which has its own path and ganglion, whereas the inferior vestibular nerve (innervating the posterior semicircular canal and the posteroinferior part of the sacculus) is most often spared, leading to a selective superior vestibular neuritis or superior division acute unilateral vestibulopathy (**Fig. 1**). These findings were supported by measurements of the function of individual semicircular canals with the HIT and the scleral coil technique[16]; this has 2-fold implications: first, with respect to clinical findings, because it explains why patients with acute unilateral vestibulopathy can suffer from postinfectious benign paroxysmal positioning nystagmus of the posterior canal and second, with respect to the pathophysiology and cause because any mechanistic theory must cohere with this fact. This common, specific pattern of involvement is supportive evidence that the typical lesion in acute unilateral vestibulopathy is most often in the vestibular nerve, rather than the labyrinth, per se, because this pattern would presumably not be favored with a labyrinthine lesion.

By similar methods that also included vestibular evoked potentials, the first cases of rare inferior vestibular neuritis or inferior division acute unilateral vestibulopathy were

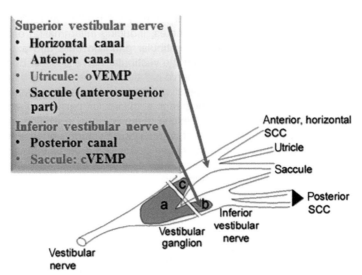

Fig. 1. Vestibular and facial nerves, the faciovestibular anastomosis, and the geniculate gan-glion. The double innervation of the posterior canal, which often leads to the preservation of its function during acute unilateral vestibulopathy, is visible. This figure also shows the innervation by the superior vestibular nerve and the inferior vestibular nerve, which ex-plains the dissociation of clinical features in superior versus inferior vestibulopathies. In the superior nerve variant, the function of the utricle is impaired, leading to reduced ocular vestibular-evoked myogenic potentials (oVEMPs). In the inferior nerve variant, the function of the saccule is impaired, leading to reduced cervical vestibular-evoked myogenic poten-tials (cVEMPs). (*Adapted from* Arbusow V, Schulz P, Strupp M, et al. Distribution of herpes simplex virus type 1 in human geniculate and vestibular ganglia: implications for vestibular neuritis. Ann Neurol 1999;46:416–9; with permission.)

described in 1996/1997.[17,18] The direction of the spontaneous nystagmus corre-sponds to the plane of the posterior canal, that is, it is contraversively torsional (pole at the 12-o'clock position of the eye beating toward the ear opposite the lesion side) with a downward component (the direction opposite to classical posterior canal BPPV). As a consequence of this atypical nystagmus pattern, it may be misdiagnosed as central (ie, located in the central nervous system rather than vestibular periphery).

If the superior and inferior vestibular nerves (total acute unilateral vestibulopathy) are both affected, horizontal nystagmus with torsional nystagmus is found with no vertical component because both vertical canals are affected. Unlike superior or inferior divi-sion vestibulopathies, this eye movement pattern cannot readily differentiate vestib-ular nerve from direct labyrinthine involvement. The presence of comorbid auditory symptoms (eg, acute unilateral hearing loss or persistent tinnitus) has clinically been used to differentiate labyrinthitis (with hearing loss) from neuritis (without hearing loss). However, this clinical distinction is of dubious anatomic value, because well-studied cases with eye movements suggest inferior division vestibular nerve involve-ment may be associated with hearing loss.

DEFINITIONS AND DIAGNOSTIC CRITERIA, BEDSIDE AND LABORATORY DIAGNOSTIC TESTS

The term acute unilateral vestibulopathy is preferred to vestibular neuritis and is used in the International Classification of Vestibular Disorders. Acute unilateral vestibulopathy is defined by the patient history and the clinical examination and, in unclear cases, laboratory examinations. It is always a diagnosis of exclusion of other disorders, in particular due to central vestibular lesions affecting the brainstem or cerebellum. When hearing loss is present, the term acute unilateral cochleovestibulopathy is preferred to the more commonly used term labyrinthitis except in cases with demonstrable labyrinthine involvement (eg, with labyrinthine extension of a bacterial middle ear infection). The less common term sudden sensorineural hearing loss with vertigo is also nonpreferred. Regardless of naming conventions, hearing loss may be encountered in otherwise typical cases of vestibular neuritis. Additional aspects of differential diagnosis related to presence of auditory symptoms are described further.

The key symptoms of acute unilateral vestibulopathy are (1) sustained rotatory vertigo, (2) apparent movement of the visual surroundings (external vertigo), (3) gait and postural unsteadiness with a tendency to fall toward the side of the affected ear, and (4) nausea and vomiting (**Fig. 2**). All these symptoms follow a monophasic illness pattern, with an acute or subacute onset and lasting generally for several days up to a few weeks. There are no typical antecedent triggers or prodromal symptoms, except for occasional spells of vertigo a few days before acute onset in a minority of patients. The presence of a recent history of viral infection is of unknown significance, as no well-designed studies have compared the frequency of recent viral infection to that of a suitable control population. To make the diagnosis, disorders affecting the brainstem or cerebellum, such as acute stroke, must be excluded. Therefore, it is important that the patient be explicitly asked about neurologic symptoms that may arise from the brainstem or cerebellum.

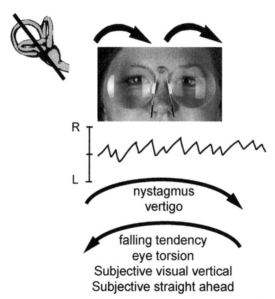

Fig. 2. Ocular signs, perception (vertigo, subjective visual vertical, and subjective straight ahead), and posture in the acute stage of right-sided acute unilateral vestibulopathy. Spontaneous vestibular nystagmus is typically horizontal-rotatory away from the side of the lesion (best observed with Frenzel or M glasses[19]). The initial perception of apparent body motion (vertigo) is also directed away from the side of the lesion, whereas measurable destabilization (Romberg fall) is typically toward the side of the lesion. The latter is the compensatory vestibulospinal reaction to the apparent tilt.

Key signs (see **Fig. 2**) of acute unilateral vestibulopathy include the following:

1. Dominantly horizontal-rotatory spontaneous nystagmus beating toward the nonaffected ear with a torsional component (beating with the pole at the 12-o'clock position directed toward the nonaffected ear); there is a variable vertical component (directed upward in cases demonstrating the superior division pattern). This peripheral vestibular spontaneous nystagmus is typically reduced in amplitude by visual fixation, as long as the relevant central structures in the brainstem and cerebellum responsible for smooth pursuit (ie, mainly the flocculus/paraflocculus and related pathways) are intact. The intensity of spontaneous nystagmus is enhanced by eye closure (one can see the nystagmus increase when examining the impression of the cornea moving behind closed lids or feel it when touching the lids gently with the tips of the fingers). It is also enhanced by visual Frenzel goggles (+16 diopters), M glasses,[19] or occlusive techniques, such as occlusive ophthalmoscopy or the penlight cover test. From a clinical point of view, this means that if there are no significant differences in the intensity of spontaneous nystagmus between with and without fixation (typical for a fixation nystagmus), this indicates a central origin and lesion and excludes acute unilateral peripheral vestibulopathy. The converse, however, is not necessarily true, because central lesions (generally those not affecting the flocculus/paraflocculus) have nystagmus that is suppressed by visual fixation. The nystagmus obeys Alexander's law, so nystagmus intensity (amplitude × frequency, which parallels slow-phase velocity) is increased with gaze shifts toward the direction of the fast phase and decreased with gaze shifts toward the direction of the slow phase of the nystagmus. This condition may mimic unilateral gaze-evoked nystagmus in a patient with mild to moderate spontaneous nystagmus that is completely suppressed by visual fixation in the primary gaze position (ie, straight ahead) but incompletely suppressed (ie, present despite visual fixation) with gaze directed toward the fast phase

2. Pathologic tilting of the subjective visual vertical (SVV) toward the affected ear; SVV tilts are associated with the pathologic ocular tilt reaction triad (bilateral ocular fundus torsion [ocular counterroll], skew deviation, and compensatory head tilt) that may be seen with peripheral vestibular lesions; an ocular tilt reaction indicates a vestibular tone imbalance in the roll plane induced by involvement of one or both vertical semicircular canals, otolith function, or both. Nowadays a simple bedside device, the so-called bucket test,[20] can be used to easily measure the SVV, which is the most sensitive parameter for an acute lesion of the vestibular system. Although assumed, patients with acute unilateral vestibulopathy of the vestibular neuritis type usually do not have a skew deviation.[21,22] Instead, clinically demonstrable vertical strabismus (skew deviation) more often indicates vestibular pseudoneuritis[21] as seen with central lesions caused by stroke or multiple sclerosis. It is likely that clinically evident skew deviations are more common in patients with complete peripheral deafferentation affecting the superior and inferior vestibular nerves, as occurs with iatrogenic lesions (vestibular neurectomy or labyrinthectomy) or sometimes in herpes zoster oticus

3. A pathologic HIT of VOR function toward the affected side and in the planes of any affected canals (horizontal and anterior > posterior); if the results of the beside HIT are unclear, a vHIT may be necessary

4. Postural unsteadiness with Romberg fall toward the affected ear

5. Ocular motor evaluation reveals, in addition to the above-mentioned signs, an apparent horizontal saccadic pursuit away from the affected side due to the spontaneous nystagmus and absence of gaze-evoked/direction-changing nystagmus with gaze toward the affected ear

Laboratory Diagnostic Tests

Caloric testing

One diagnostic marker of acute unilateral vestibulopathy is a peripheral vestibular deficit on the affected side. Caloric testing typically shows hyporesponsiveness or unresponsiveness of the tested and affected horizontal canal (it tests, however, only the VOR in the low-frequency range of about 0.003 Hz). Because there is also a large intersubject variability of the nystagmus induced by caloric irrigation and a small intraindividual variability of the response of the right and the left labyrinths in healthy subjects, Jongkees's formula for vestibular paresis,[23] $(((R30° + R44°) - (L30° + L44°))/(R30° + R44° + L30° + L44°)) \times 100$, should be used to determine its presence. In this formula, for instance, R30° is the mean peak slow phase velocity during caloric irrigation with 30°C water. Vestibular paresis is usually defined as greater than 25% asymmetry between the 2 sides. This formula allows a direct comparison of the function of the horizontal semicircular canals of both labyrinths, which is important because of the large interindividual variability of caloric excitability. Caloric testing is typically normal in inferior division patterns (inferior vestibular neuritis).

Video head-impulse test

Because the bedside HIT is not always reliable (eg, because of covert refixation saccades during the HIT head rotation), examination of patients with the vHIT is recommended to diagnose a high frequency of the VOR, to examine all 3 canals, and to differentiate between a peripheral and central vestibular lesion.[24,25] In terms of a 3-dimensional analysis, superior division, inferior division, and total unilateral vestibulopathy patterns can thus be diagnosed and differentiated; in superior division forms, the function of the posterior canal is spared; in inferior vestibular neuritis, the function of the horizontal and anterior canal is spared.

Cervical and ocular vestibular-evoked myogenic potentials

cVEMPs can be recorded from the sternocleidomastoid muscles using an audible click stimulus. There is evidence that cVEMPs originate in the medial (striola) area of the saccular macula. Therefore, cVEMPs allow examination of the function of the saccule and, thereby, of the inferior vestibular nerve (see Refs.[26,27]). cVEMPs are preserved in at least two-thirds of the patients with acute unilateral vestibulopathy,[28] which is typical of superior vestibular nerve involvement because the inferior part of the vestibular nerve is spared in most patients and it supplies the saccule and posterior canal. In contrast, in inferior and total vestibular nerve involvement, the cVEMPs are reduced or absent, indicating impaired saccular function.[26,27]

Intense air-conducted sound and bone-conducted vibration can elicit oVEMPs (see Refs.[26,27]). In patients with superior or total vestibular nerve involvement, the amplitude of the oVEMPs is typically reduced or absent, suggesting disruption of utricular afferents, presumably within the superior vestibular nerve.

Differential Diagnosis and Other Clinical Problems

Central nervous system dysfunctions or lesions in the lower brainstem or cerebellum (**Fig. 3**) may mimic acute unilateral vestibulopathy (so-called vestibular pseudoneuritis), as can other peripheral vestibular disorders. There is no single, pathognomonic clinical sign or laboratory test to confirm an acute unilateral vestibulopathy. Therefore, the diagnosis ultimately rests on a combination of clinical features consistent with the disorder and reasonable exclusion of mimics.

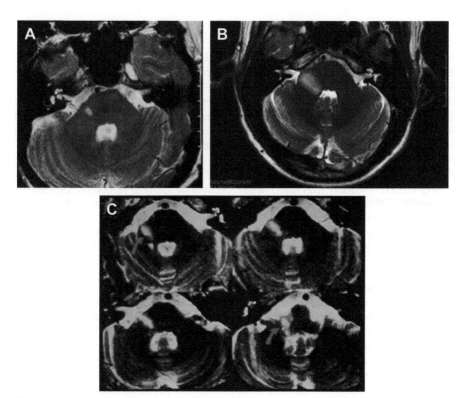

Fig. 3. Fascicular and nuclear lesion of the vestibular nerve due to (*A*) an plaque in mutiple sclerosis (*B*) brainstem encephalitis (*B*), and (*C*) vascular lesion mimicking vestibular neuritis (T2-weighted magnetic resonance images, *red arrows* indicate infartion).

Central lesions mimicking acute unilateral vestibulopathy

The most common topographic locations for central lesions causing acute monophasic illnesses similar to peripheral acute unilateral vestibulopathy are in the lateral medulla, lateral pons, or inferior cerebellum. The vascular territories most often involved are the posterior inferior cerebellar artery (PICA) and anterior inferior cerebellar artery (AICA), although lesions in the superior cerebellar artery territory can sometimes produce a similar syndrome. The structures most often involved are the inferior cerebellar peduncle, medial vestibular nucleus, and nodulus, although other structures have also been implicated.

Brainstem lesions in the lateral medulla or pons affecting the root entry zone of the vestibular nerve or the medial and superior VN may be confused with lesions of the peripheral vestibular nerve or labyrinths. The authors have seen several patients with multiple sclerosis who have pontomedullary plaques or small lacunar strokes[29] at the root entry zone of the eighth nerve, which leads to a fascicular nerve lesion, which mimics acute unilateral vestibulopathy, vestibular pseudoneuritis. A small lacunar infarction of the VN[30] or the dorsolateral pons may also mimic acute unilateral vestibulopathy.

If the patient has obvious additional brainstem signs, the differential diagnosis between central and peripheral causes of unilateral vestibular loss is simple. When this is not the case, distinguishing central from peripheral disorders is difficult. Several studies have examined ocular motor and related signs as a means to differentiate acute unilateral vestibulopathy from central vestibular pseudoneuritis and the final diagnosis was assessed by neuroimaging.[21,22,31,32] No single sign (HIT, saccadic pursuit, gaze-evoked nystagmus, SVV) is sufficient to identify all cases of stroke. In most studies, however, skew deviation or a normal result on HIT in a patient with acute onset of vertigo and nystagmus was a specific (albeit nonsensitive) sign for vestibular pseudoneuritis.[21,22,31] A combination of the above-mentioned clinical signs, however, increases the sensitivity and specificity to more than 90%[21,22,31,32] besting the accuracy of other bedside methods, including even MRI neuroimaging in the early acute disease state.

Cerebellar infarction in the PICA territory may also mimic acute unilateral vestibulopathy,[33–36] especially if it is an isolated nodular infarction.[37] It may also cause an incomplete ocular tilt reaction,[38] in particular, if the dentate nucleus is involved.[39] Cerebellar infarction in AICA territory may also mimic acute unilateral vestibulopathy closely and sometimes causes an abnormal head impulse VOR either by involvement of the flocculus or, in some cases, through labyrinthine infarction. However, it is most often associated with unilateral hearing loss (due to cochlear ischemia) or additional brainstem signs. Thus, clinical examination and testing of hearing generally allow differentiation between acute unilateral vestibulopathy and vestibular pseudoneuritis.

Vestibular migraine attacks, which are presumably often central in localization (but without causing overt structural lesions), may also mimic acute unilateral vestibulopathy because they may be associated with spinning vertigo and horizontal-torsional nystagmus. Accompanying symptoms and the course of the disease help to differentiate between the 2 entities. Most vestibular migraine attacks abate within 24 to 72 hours after onset, unlike most cases of acute unilateral vestibulopathy.

Peripheral vestibular lesions
The differential diagnosis of peripheral labyrinthine and vestibular nerve disorders mimicking acute unilateral vestibulopathy includes numerous uncommon and rare conditions. Nevertheless, extensive laboratory examinations, lumbar puncture, and computed tomography/MRI are not part of the routine diagnosis of acute unilateral vestibulopathy for 2 reasons: (1) the rarity of these disorders and (2) typical additional signs and symptoms indicative of other disorders. An initial monosymptomatic vertigo attack in Menière's disease or a short attack in vestibular paroxysmia can be confused with acute unilateral vestibulopathy in a patient admitted to the hospital during the acute stage. The shortness of the attack and the patient's rapid recovery, however, allow differentiation. During the course of the disease, almost all patients with Menière's disease develop hypoacusis, tinnitus, or aural fullness in the affected ear, which also allows differentiation.

An initially burning pain and blisters as well as hearing disorders and facial paresis are typical for herpes zoster oticus (Ramsay Hunt syndrome) (in such cases, acyclovir or valacyclovir is indicated). There may be a skew deviation in herpes zoster oticus due to the complete unilateral peripheral vestibular deficit, that is, of the superior and inferior parts of the vestibular nerve and, contrary to typical cases of acute unilateral vestibulopathy, a contrast enhancement of the eighth cranial nerve. Cogan syndrome (often overlooked) is a severe autoimmune disease accompanied by interstitial keratitis and audiovestibular symptoms (hearing disorders are prominent). It occurs most often in young adults and responds, in part only temporarily, to the early administration of high doses of corticosteroids (1000 mg/d for 3–5 days, then slowly tapered off) or, like other autoimmune diseases of the inner ear, to a combination of steroids and cyclophosphamide.

The labyrinth may be affected by an infection by direct spread of infection (usually from the middle ear) or by toxins or inflammatory responses to either of these. This condition has been further characterized as either a purulent or a serous labyrinthitis.

The former suggests a purulent invasion of the membranous labyrinth with bacteria and macrophages, the latter a response to toxic or inflammatory mediators. An infection can spread to the inner ear by one of the following routes: (1) direct invasion from the middle ear, as with otitis media or cholesteatomas; (2) indirect invasion by way of cerebrospinal fluid communicating with the perilymphatic fluid, as with meningitis; (3) hematogenous spread via circulating microorganisms in the blood stream; (4) neurogenic spread as with neurotropic viruses. Autoimmune and toxic effects may also induce an inflammation of the labyrinth that can be termed labyrinthitis. However, such maladies generally have a slow course, and symptoms develop less acutely. The symptoms of labyrinthitis mimic those of any disorder that affects the inner ear, that is, hearing loss, dizziness/vertigo, and tinnitus. However, if such symptoms present together or within a short time frame with signs of middle ear or temporal bone infections, one should strongly suspect an infectious spread to the labyrinth.

Suspected labyrinthine symptoms (hearing loss, dizziness, tinnitus) combined with signs of ear infection must be presumed to result from bacterial labyrinthitis and require immediate treatment. Left untreated, labyrinthitis may cause permanent inner ear damage, including the potential for complete deafness as well as complete loss of balance function in that ear. Even after recovery, secondary balance disturbances (delayed hydrops) may produce a secondary Menière's syndrome clinical picture. An even greater danger is that labyrinthitis from direct middle ear invasion may quickly spread to the intracranial space, causing meningitis (ie, otogenic meningitis). Otogenic meningitis is life threatening and may have a fulminant course requiring emergency treatment to prevent death or permanent disability.

Vestibular schwannomas, which arise in the myelin sheaths of the vestibular part of the eighth nerve, normally present with unilateral tinnitus or hearing loss rather than vertigo. The primary symptom is a slowly progressive unilateral reduction of hearing without any identifiable otologic cause. This reduction is combined with a caloric hypoexcitability or nonexcitability. Under normal circumstances, they only cause vertigo, a tendency to fall, and nystagmus if the pontomedullary brainstem and the flocculus are compressed. Rarely, acute vertigo may occur in cases of a purely intracanalicular dilatation, which can be confirmed by MRI and treated early by microsurgery or using gamma knife radiotherapy.

SHORT-TERM TREATMENT OPTIONS (INCLUDING MANIPULATIVE, PHARMACOLOGIC, REHABILITATIVE)

The management of acute unilateral vestibulopathy involves (1) symptomatic treatment with antivertiginous drugs (eg, meclizine, dimenhydrinate, scopolamine, or in severe cases benzodiazepines) to attenuate vertigo, dizziness, and nausea/vomiting; (2) causal treatment with corticosteroids to improve recovery of peripheral vestibular function; and (3) physical therapy (vestibular exercises and balance training) to improve central vestibular compensation.

Symptomatic Treatment and Improvement of Central Compensation

To treat nausea and vomiting in acute unilateral vestibulopathy, drugs such as dimenhydrinate (100–300 mg/d) or in severe cases even benzodiazepines can be given. Because they are sedatives and may delay or reduce central compensation of the vestibular tone imbalance between the 2 labyrinths, these agents should not be administered for more than 3 days. This clinical recommendation has generally been made largely on theoretic grounds, but animal studies have begun to provide supporting evidence for this approach.

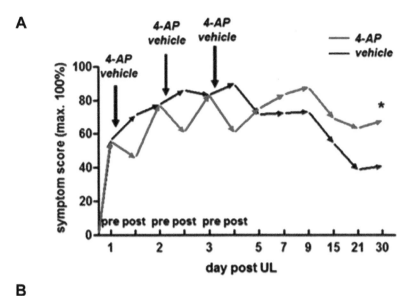

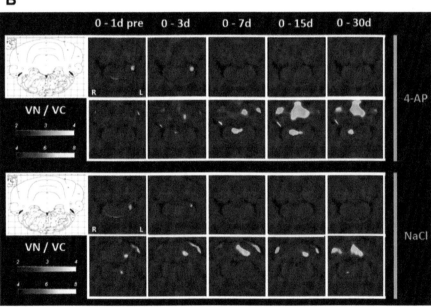

Fig. 4. Effects of 4-aminopyridine (4-AP) on behavioral symptoms in acute vestibulopathy/ acute unilateral lesion (UL) and central vestibular compensation. (A) Postural asymmetry was transiently decreased by 4-AP after administration on days 1, 2, and 3 following chemical unilateral labyrinthectomy in rats. However, the postural asymmetry persisted longer in the 4-AP group compared with the vehicle group, which indicated impaired vestibular compensation. Values are depicted as percentage of maximum symptom scores. Significant differences between groups are indicated by an asterisk. (B) Sequential whole brain micro-PET with fludeoxyglucose F 18 dynamics after chemical unilateral labyrinthectomy in the 4-AP and control groups. A significant asymmetry of regional cerebral glucose metabolism (rCGM) appeared in the vestibular nuclei in the 4-AP group after day 3 (P<.001). The control group showed no changes in rCGM of the vestibular nuclei after day 3 (L, left; R, right; VC, vestibulocerebellum; VN, vestibular nuclei). (*Adapted from* Beck R, Gunther L, Xiong G, et al. The mixed blessing of treating symptoms in acute vestibular failure - evidence from a 4-aminopyridine experiment. Exp Neurol 2014;261:638–45; with permission.)

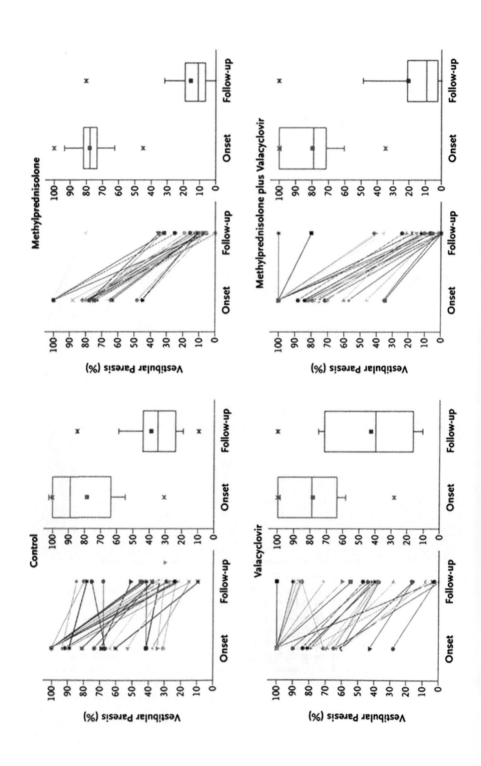

There are few animal studies on the effects of pharmacologic agents on central compensation (overview in Ref.[40]). A recent study in rats, however, indicated that 4-aminopyridine improves postural symptoms in acute vestibular failure but likely also blunts the course of subsequent vestibular compensation[41] (**Fig. 4**). This observation underscores the fact that symptomatic treatment should only be given on demand and for a short time in acute vestibular neuritis.

Acetyl-DL-leucine and betahistine have been viewed as promising substances to promote vestibular compensation.[42] However, experimental evidence on their efficacy and mechanism of action is limited (acetyl-DL-leucine: negative results in 3 randomized trials). It has not yet been sufficiently investigated whether these drugs influence central compensation in humans and, if so, to what extent. To further evaluate these issues, there is an on-going clinical trial on the effects of betahistine on central compensation in acute unilateral vestibulopathy (betahistine-dihydrochloride, 48 mg thrice a day, vs placebo; the BETAVEST trial), which focuses on postural imbalance, spontaneous nystagmus, and functional impairment.

Available evidence suggests one should carefully consider the goals of pharmacotherapy in acute unilateral vestibulopathy before proceeding. Because a symptomatic therapy most often decreases the vestibular tone imbalance (which drives central compensation), it likely has a negative impact on central compensation and the long-term outcome. This result further supports the use of vestibular exercises[43,44] that should increase vestibular tone imbalance in particular by head-movements, leading to increased central compensation.

Causative Treatment

In a randomized controlled trial, it was shown by caloric irrigation that monotherapy with steroids (methylprednisolone, 100 mg/d) significantly improved the recovery of peripheral vestibular function in acute unilateral vestibulopathy (**Fig. 5**).[45] These findings are supported by both a meta-analysis[46] and an observational study.[47] A more recent single-blinded trial that compared corticosteroids to vestibular exercises in acute unilateral vestibulopathy found that vestibular exercises are as effective as treatment with corticosteroids in clinical, caloric, and otolith recovery[48]; corticosteroid therapy seems to enhance earlier complete acute unilateral vestibulopathy resolution, with no added benefit in the long-term clinical prognosis. In agreement with these

◄───

Fig. 5. Effects of steroids and a virostatic agent on recovery of vestibular function. Unilateral vestibular failure within 3 days after symptom onset and after 12 months. Vestibular function was determined by caloric irrigation, using the vestibular paresis formula (which allows a direct comparison of the function of both labyrinths) for each patient in the placebo (*upper left*), methylprednisolone (*upper right*), valacyclovir (*lower right*), and methylprednisolone plus valacyclovir (*lower left*) groups. Also shown are box plot charts for each group with the mean (■) ± SD and 25% and 75% percentile (box plot), as well as the 1% and 99% range (x). A clinically relevant vestibular paresis was defined as greater than 25% asymmetry between the right-sided and the left-sided responses.[50] Follow-up examination showed that vestibular function improved in all 4 groups: in the placebo group from 78.9 ± 24.0 (mean ± SD) to 39.0 ± 19.9, in the methylprednisolone group from 78.7 ± 15.8 to 15.4 ± 16.2, in the valacyclovir group from 78.4 ± 20.0 to 42.7 ± 32.3, and in the methylprednisolone plus valacyclovir group from 78.6 ± 21.1 to 20.4 ± 28.4. Analysis of variance revealed that methylprednisolone and methylprednisolone plus valacyclovir caused significantly more improvement than placebo or valacyclovir alone. The combination of both was not superior to steroid monotherapy. (*From* Strupp M, Zingler VC, Arbusow V, et al. Methylprednisolone, valacyclovir, or the combination for vestibular neuritis. N Engl J Med 2004;351:354–61; with permission.)

findings, a Cochrane analysis[49] and a meta-analysis[46] make no general treatment recommendation for corticosteroids; they may improve only the recovery of canal paresis,[46] and their effects on life quality have not yet been investigated sufficiently. Thus, further randomized controlled trials are necessary. In clinical practice, however, 3 weeks of treatment with corticosteroids can be considered (eg, methylprednisolone, 100 mg/d, within 3 days after symptom onset; taper off by 20 mg every fourth day).[45]

Vestibular Physical Therapy

A gradual program of physical exercise under the supervision of a physiotherapist improves the central vestibular compensation of a peripheral deficit. First, static stabilization is concentrated on, and then dynamic exercises are done for balance control and gaze stabilization during eye-head-body movements. The degree of difficulty of exercises for equilibrium and balance should be successively increased more than normal levels, both with and without visual stabilization. The efficacy of physiotherapy in improving central vestibulospinal compensation in patients with acute unilateral vestibulopathy has been proved in a prospective, randomized, and controlled clinical study (**Fig. 6**)[43] and confirmed in a Cochrane review.[44]

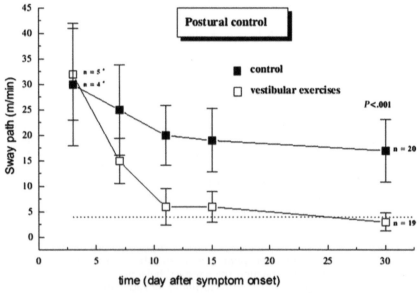

Fig. 6. Time course of the changes in total sway path (SP) values for a patient group and a control group, both after acute vestibular neuritis without recovery of the labyrinthine function. The initial values for SP (meters per minute, mean ± SD), measured with eyes closed and standing on a compliant foam rubber-padded posturography platform, were not significantly different in the 2 groups, whereas the SP values in the therapy group normalized significantly faster in the course of the study. On day 30 (statistical end point), there was a significant difference between the 2 groups (analysis of variance, $P<.001$). Thus, balance training improves the vestibulospinal compensation of an acute unilateral peripheral vestibular deficit. The dotted line indicates the normal range. (During the first days after onset of the illness, some of the patients had such pronounced disturbances of postural control that they were unable to stand on the platform for the amount of time required to perform the measurements [>10 seconds] without falling.) (*From* Strupp M, Arbusow V, Maag KP, et al. Vestibular exercises improve central vestibulospinal compensation after vestibular neuritis. Neurology 1998;51:838–44; with permission.)

SUPPLEMENTARY DATA

Supplementary data related to this article can be found online at http://dx.doi.org/10.1016/j.ncl.2015.04.012.

REFERENCES

1. Neuhauser HK. Epidemiology of vertigo. Curr Opin Neurol 2007;20:40–6.
2. Sekitani T, Imate Y, Noguchi T, et al. Vestibular neuronitis: epidemiological survey by questionnaire in Japan. Acta Otolaryngol (Stockh) Suppl 1993;503:9–12.
3. Adamec I, Krbot SM, Handzic J, et al. Incidence, seasonality and comorbidity in vestibular neuritis. Neurol Sci 2015;36:91–5.
4. Brandt T, Dieterich M, Strupp M. Vertigo and dizziness - common complaints. 2nd edition. London: Springer; 2013.
5. Gioacchini FM, Alicandri-Ciufelli M, Kaleci S, et al. Prevalence and diagnosis of vestibular disorders in children: a review. Int J Pediatr Otorhinolaryngol 2014; 78:718–24.
6. Huppert D, Strupp M, Theil D, et al. Low recurrence rate of vestibular neuritis: a long-term follow-up. Neurology 2006;67:1870–1.
7. Kim YH, Kim KS, Kim KJ, et al. Recurrence of vertigo in patients with vestibular neuritis. Acta Otolaryngol 2011;131:1172–7.
8. Strupp M, Brandt T. Vestibular neuritis. Semin Neurol 2009;29:509–19.
9. Jeong SH, Kim HJ, Kim JS. Vestibular neuritis. Semin Neurol 2013;33:185–94.
10. Arbusow V, Schulz P, Strupp M, et al. Distribution of herpes simplex virus type 1 in human geniculate and vestibular ganglia: implications for vestibular neuritis. Ann Neurol 1999;46:416–9.
11. Theil D, Derfuss T, Strupp M, et al. Cranial nerve palsies: herpes simplex virus type 1 and varizella-zoster virus latency. Ann Neurol 2002;51:273–4.
12. Gianoli G, Goebel J, Mowry S, et al. Anatomic differences in the lateral vestibular nerve channels and their implications in vestibular neuritis. Otol Neurotol 2005;26: 489–94.
13. Arbusow V, Theil D, Schulz P, et al. Distribution of HSV-1 in human geniculate and vestibular ganglia: implications for vestibular neuritis. Ann N Y Acad Sci 2003; 1004:409–13.
14. Fetter M, Dichgans J. Vestibular neuritis spares the inferior division of the vestibular nerve. Brain 1996;119:755–63.
15. Büchele W, Brandt T. Vestibular neuritis–a horizontal semicircular canal paresis? Adv Otorhinolaryngol 1988;42:157–61.
16. Fetter M, Dichgans J. Three-dimensional human VOR in acute vestibular lesions. Ann N Y Acad Sci 1996;781:619–21.
17. Bohmer A, Straumann D, Fetter M. Three-dimensional analysis of spontaneous nystagmus in peripheral vestibular lesions. Ann Otol Rhinol Laryngol 1997;106:61–8.
18. Murofushi T, Halmagyi GM, Yavor RA, et al. Absent vestibular evoked myogenic potentials in vestibular neurolabyrinthitis. An indicator of inferior vestibular nerve involvement? Arch Otolaryngol Head Neck Surg 1996;122:845–8.
19. Strupp M, Fischer C, Hanss L, et al. The takeaway Frenzel goggles: a Fresnel-based device. Neurology 2014;83:1241–5.
20. Zwergal A, Rettinger N, Frenzel C, et al. A bucket of static vestibular function. Neurology 2009;72:1689–92.
21. Cnyrim CD, Newman-Toker D, Karch C, et al. Bedside differentiation of vestibular neuritis from central "vestibular pseudoneuritis". J Neurol Neurosurg Psychiatry 2008;79:458–60.

22. Kattah JC, Talkad AV, Wang DZ, et al. HINTS to diagnose stroke in the acute vestibular syndrome: three-step bedside oculomotor examination more sensitive than early MRI diffusion-weighted imaging. Stroke 2009;40:3504–10.

23. Jongkees LB, Maas J, Philipszoon A. Clinical electronystagmography: a detailed study of electronystagmography in 341 patients with vertigo. Pract Otorhinolaryngol (Basel) 1962;24:65–93.

24. Chen L, Todd M, Halmagyi GM, et al. Head impulse gain and saccade analysis in pontine-cerebellar stroke and vestibular neuritis. Neurology 2014;83:1513–22.

25. Mantokoudis G, Saber Tehrani AS, Wozniak A, et al. VOR gain by head impulse video-oculography differentiates acute vestibular neuritis from stroke. Otol Neurotol 2014;36:457–65.

26. Rosengren SM, Kingma H. New perspectives on vestibular evoked myogenic potentials. Curr Opin Neurol 2013;26:74–80.

27. Curthoys IS. The interpretation of clinical tests of peripheral vestibular function. Laryngoscope 2012;122:1342–52.

28. Manzari L, Burgess AM, MacDougall HG, et al. Vestibular function after vestibular neuritis. Int J Audiol 2013;52:713–8.

29. Thomke F, Hopf HC. Pontine lesions mimicking acute peripheral vestibulopathy. J Neurol Neurosurg Psychiatry 1999;66:340–9.

30. Kim HA, Lee H. Isolated vestibular nucleus infarction mimicking acute peripheral vestibulopathy. Stroke 2010;41:1558–60.

31. Newman-Toker DE, Kattah JC, Alvernia JE, et al. Normal head impulse test differentiates acute cerebellar strokes from vestibular neuritis. Neurology 2008;70:2378–85.

32. Chen L, Lee W, Chambers BR, et al. Diagnostic accuracy of acute vestibular syndrome at the bedside in a stroke unit. J Neurol 2011;258:855–61.

33. Duncan GW, Parker SW, Fisher CM. Acute cerebellar infarction in the PICA territory. Arch Neurol 1975;32:364–8.

34. Huang CY, Yu YL. Small cerebellar strokes may mimic labyrinthine lesions. J Neurol Neurosurg Psychiatry 1985;48:263–5.

35. Magnusson M, Norrving B. Cerebellar infarctions as the cause of 'vestibular neuritis'. Acta Otolaryngol Suppl 1991;481:258–9.

36. Magnusson M, Norrving B. Cerebellar infarctions and 'vestibular neuritis'. Acta Otolaryngol Suppl 1993;503:64–6.

37. Moon IS, Kim JS, Choi KD, et al. Isolated nodular infarction. Stroke 2009;40:487–91.

38. Mossman S, Halmagyi GM. Partial ocular tilt reaction due to unilateral cerebellar lesion. Neurology 2000;49:491–3.

39. Baier B, Bense S, Dieterich M. Are signs of ocular tilt reaction in patients with cerebellar lesions mediated by the dentate nucleus? Brain 2008;131:1445–54.

40. Dutia MB. Mechanisms of vestibular compensation: recent advances. Curr Opin Otolaryngol Head Neck Surg 2010;18:420–4.

41. Beck R, Gunther L, Xiong G, et al. The mixed blessing of treating symptoms in acute vestibular failure - evidence from a 4-aminopyridine experiment. Exp Neurol 2014;261:638–45.

42. Gunther L, Beck R, Xiong G, et al. N-acetyl-L-leucine accelerates vestibular compensation after unilateral labyrinthectomy by action in the cerebellum and thalamus. PLoS One 2015;10:e0120891.

43. Strupp M, Arbusow V, Maag KP, et al. Vestibular exercises improve central vestibulospinal compensation after vestibular neuritis. Neurology 1998;51:838–44.

44. McDonnell MN, Hillier SL. Vestibular rehabilitation for unilateral peripheral vestibular dysfunction. Cochrane Database Syst Rev 2015;(1):CD005397.

45. Strupp M, Zingler VC, Arbusow V, et al. Methylprednisolone, valacyclovir, or the combination for vestibular neuritis. N Engl J Med 2004;351:354–61.

46. Goudakos JK, Markou KD, Franco-Vidal V, et al. Corticosteroids in the treatment of vestibular neuritis: a systematic review and meta-analysis. Otol Neurotol 2010; 31:183–9.

47. Karlberg ML, Magnusson M. Treatment of acute vestibular neuronitis with glucocorticoids. Otol Neurotol 2011;32:1140–3.

48. Goudakos JK, Markou KD, Psillas G, et al. Corticosteroids and vestibular exercises in vestibular neuritis. Single-blind randomized clinical trial. JAMA Otolaryngol Head Neck Surg 2014;140:434–40.

49. Fishman JM, Burgess C, Waddell A. Corticosteroids for the treatment of idiopathic acute vestibular dysfunction (vestibular neuritis). Cochrane Database Syst Rev 2011;(5):CD008607.

50. Honrubia V. Quantitative vestibular function tests and the clinical examination. In: Herdman SJ, editor. Vestibular rehabilitation. 1st edition. Philadelphia: F.A. Davis; 1994. p. 113–64.

Acute Diagnosis and Management of Stroke Presenting Dizziness or Vertigo

CrossMark

Seung-Han Lee, MD, PhD[a], Ji-Soo Kim, MD, PhD[b],*

KEYWORDS

- Stroke • Vertigo • Nystagmus • Head impulse test • Cerebellum • Brainstem

KEY POINTS

- Stroke is an important cause of acute dizziness/vertigo in the emergency department.
- Small stroke involving the cerebellum and brainstem may cause acute vestibular syndrome in isolation.
- Findings of bedside neuro-otologic examinations including direction-changing nystagmus and negative head impulse test are useful for differentiating stroke from a more benign inner ear disorder.
- Neuroimaging studies, including diffusion MRI, may fail to disclose small strokes in the posterior fossa, especially during the acute stage.

 Video of head impulse tests accompanies this article at http://www.neurologic. theclinics.com/

CASE (WALLENBERG SYNDROME)

A 55-year-old man with hypertension presented with acute vertigo and unsteadiness for 2 days. He reported a sensation of spinning and being pushed rightward to the ground. He also had nausea and blurred vision, but denied hearing loss or tinnitus.

The blood pressure measured 160/100 mm Hg. He showed spontaneous left-beating nystagmus that increased with removal of visual fixation and during leftward gaze, and changed into right-beating nystagmus during rightward gaze. After horizontal head shaking for about 15 seconds, the nystagmus changed into right-beating nystagmus. Saccades were hypermetric

[a] Department of Neurology, Chonnam National University Medical School, Gwangju, Korea;
[b] Department of Neurology, Seoul National University Bundang Hospital, Seoul National University College Medicine, Seoul, Korea
* Corresponding author. Department of Neurology, Seoul National University Bundang Hospital, Seoul National University College of Medicine, 173-82 Gumi-ro, Bundang-gu, Seongnam-si, Gyeonggi-do 463-707, Korea.
E-mail address: jisookim@snu.ac.kr

Neurol Clin 33 (2015) 687–698
http://dx.doi.org/10.1016/j.ncl.2015.04.006
0733-8619/15/$ – see front matter © 2015 Elsevier Inc. All rights reserved.

neurologic.theclinics.com

to the right and hypometric to the left, which was consistent with rightward saccadic lateropulsion. Leftward smooth pursuit was impaired. Head impulse tests (HITs) were normal (Video 1). The gag reflex was diminished. He also showed right Horner syndrome, and diminished pain and temperature sensation on the right side of the face and left side of the body. Right upper extremity was dysmetric on finger-to-nose testing. He fell to the right on standing.

The clinical features were consistent with acute prolonged vertigo syndrome. Given the Horner syndrome, direction-changing gaze-evoked nystagmus (GEN), central-type head-shaking nystagmus (HSN), normal HITs, crossed sensory loss, and severe imbalance, he had a clinical diagnosis of Wallenberg syndrome, and MRIs confirmed an acute infarction in the territory of right posterior inferior cerebellar artery (PICA) involving the right lateral medulla and inferior cerebellum (**Fig. 1**).

PREVALENCE AND PATHOMECHANISM

Strokes may present as acute dizziness/vertigo.[1] Vascular vertigo mostly presents as acute (AVS, acute prolonged dizziness) or episodic (EVS, spontaneous recurrent dizziness) vestibular syndrome, and rarely positional vestibular syndrome (recurrent positional dizziness). Approximately 20% of ischemic strokes occur in the territory of the posterior (vertebrobasilar) circulation, and dizziness/vertigo is the most common symptom of vertebrobasilar ischemia.[2] Even though it has been a medical adage that isolated dizziness/vertigo is rare, if any, in central lesions including strokes,[2] inferior cerebellar and small brainstem infarctions have been increasingly recognized as a cause of isolated vertigo with improvements in clinical neurotology and neuroimaging.[3]

It is important to differentiate isolated vertigo of a vascular cause from more benign disorders involving the inner ear, as managements and prognosis differ between those conditions.[4,5] Misdiagnosis of acute stroke can result in significant morbidity and mortality, whereas overdiagnosis of vascular vertigo leads to unnecessary workups and medication.[4] Stroke is a small (3.2%) proportion of all dizziness presentations to the emergency department (ED).[6] However, ED patients with dizziness/vertigo had a twofold higher risk of stroke or cardiovascular events than those without during a follow-up of 3 years.[7] Furthermore, those who had been hospitalized with isolated vertigo had a threefold higher risk for stroke than the general population during the 4-year follow-up.[8] Particularly, the patients with 3 or more risk factors had a 5.5-fold higher risk for stroke than those without risk factors.[8]

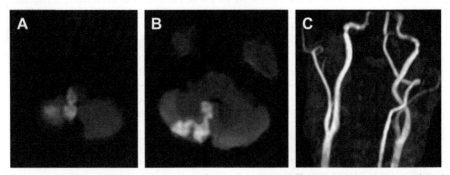

Fig. 1. Brain MRI and MR angiography of the case. Axial diffusion-weighted images (*A*, *B*) show acute infarctions involving the lateral medulla, and infero-medial cerebellum including the nodulus and tonsil on the right side. The right vertebral artery is not visualized on MR angiography (*C*).

Stroke Presenting with Acute Vestibular Syndrome

AVS constitutes approximately 10% to 20% of ED dizziness, so is responsible for approximately 400,000 to 800,000 US ED visits annually.[9] It is estimated that approximately 25% of AVS cases are due to stroke.[10] Most patients with dizziness/vertigo from ischemic strokes develop AVS, but only approximately 20% have focal neurologic signs, whereas the remainder have isolated AVS.[10,11]

Strokes presenting with AVS may occur all along the vestibular pathways from the inner ear to cerebral hemisphere, but mostly involve the structures supplied by the posterior circulation (**Fig. 2**).[5]

DIAGNOSIS AND CLASSIFICATION OF STROKES

Vascular vertigo should be a prime suspicion in patients with AVS and vascular risk factors even though confirmation of a stroke is mostly based on the findings of neurotological examination and imaging of the brain, including the blood vessels. Vascular causes should be suspected in EVS, especially when the dizzy spells last only minutes in patients with stroke risk factors. Vascular vertigo may be classified according to the presentation (prolonged vs episodic), involved vascular territories, and underlying etiologies. Brain imaging assists in determining the involved territories and causes of the strokes. Ischemic strokes account for approximately 80% of all cases.[12] This article covers only the vascular vertigo due to infarctions involving the cerebellum and medulla.

Cerebellar Infarction

The cerebellum is supplied by 3 arteries: the PICA, anterior inferior cerebellar artery (AICA), and superior cerebellar artery (SCA). In contrast to the traditional belief, the well-known cerebellar signs, such as dysarthria and dysmetria, are frequently absent in circumscribed cerebellar infarctions.[13] Thus, the findings of detailed ocular motor examinations are important in diagnosing cerebellar infarction, the most common cause of isolated vascular vertigo (**Table 1**).[14]

Posterior inferior cerebellar artery infarction

PICA territory infarction is the most common cause of isolated AVS. In a previous study, 25 of 240 patients with isolated cerebellar infarction developed isolated vertigo and 24 of them had isolated vertigo from an infarction in the territory of the medial PICA.[13] A more recent study using diffusion-weighted images found that 75% of patients with at least one vascular risk factor and isolated AVS had acute stroke, mostly involving the caudal cerebellum in the medial PICA territory.[15]

The unidirectional spontaneous nystagmus and mild imbalance observed in some patients with PICA territory infarction are similar to those in acute peripheral vestibulopathy.[14] However, normal HITs with or without GEN almost always permit differentiation of PICA territory cerebellar infarction from acute peripheral vestibulopathy.[15]

The nodulus participates in controlling eye movements and in postural adjustments to gravity, and receives blood supply from the medial PICA.[16] Patients with isolated nodular infarctions present with isolated vertigo and moderate to severe imbalance. The most common manifestation is unidirectional spontaneous nystagmus and falling in the opposite direction, which mimics peripheral vestibulopathy. The direction of spontaneous nystagmus is uniformly ipsilesional in unilateral lesions. However, the HITs and bithermal caloric tests are normal. Other findings include periodic alternating nystagmus, perverted HSN, paroxysmal positional nystagmus, and impaired tilt suppression of the postrotatory nystagmus.[16]

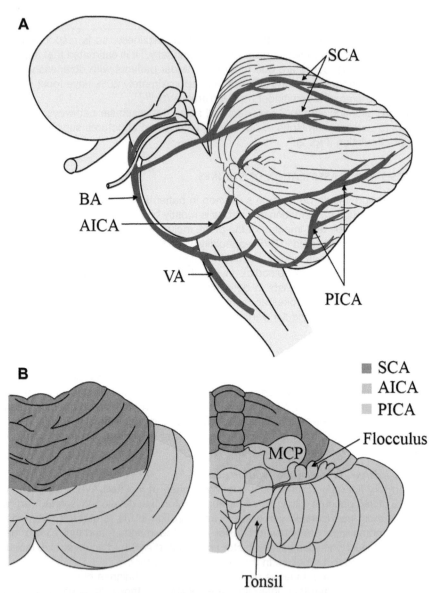

Fig. 2. The cerebrovascular anatomy of the posterior circulation (*A*) and vascular territory of the cerebellum (*B*). The cerebellum receives its blood supply from 3 paired arteries. The PICA usually derives from the distal vertebral artery. The AICA usually branches from the proximal or mid-basilar artery, and the SCA usually stems from the distal basilar artery. In general, shorter, proximal branches from all 3 of the cerebellar arteries supply portions of the brainstem, whereas longer circumferential branches supply the cerebellum proper. Variations are common. BA, basilar artery; VA, vertebral artery.

Tonsilar infarction may be a cause of acute vestibular syndrome. In a previous study, a patient with unilateral tonsilar infarction showed (1) nearly completely abolished ipsilateral smooth pursuit and impaired contralateral pursuit, (2) a low-amplitude ipsilesional spontaneous nystagmus without fixation, (3) gaze-holding

Table 1
Characteristics of cerebellar infarctions causing acute vestibular syndrome

Features	Posterior Inferior Cerebellar Artery	Anterior Inferior Cerebellar Artery	Superior Cerebellar Artery
Typical origin	Vertebral artery	Proximal or mid-basilar artery	Distal basilar artery
Major branches	Medial branch, lateral branch	Cerebellar branches, internal auditory artery	Medial branch, lateral branch
Key brainstem structures supplied by proximal branches	Posterolateral medulla: cranial nerve nuclei (V, VIII [vestibular], IX, X) and fascicles (IX, X), sympathetic tract, spinothalamic tract, inferior cerebellar peduncle	Posterolateral pons: cranial nerve nuclei (V, VII, VIII [vestibular, cochlear]) and fascicles (VII, VIII), sympathetic tract, spinothalamic tract, middle cerebellar peduncle	Posterolateral midbrain (and upper lateral pons): cranial nerve nuclei (IV, V) and fascicle (IV), sympathetic tract, spinothalamic tract, medial lemniscus, superior cerebellar peduncle
Cerebellar and distal structures supplied by major branches	Posteroinferior cerebellum, including inferior vermis (including uvula, nodulus), paraflocculus	Anteroinferior cerebellum, including flocculus. Inner ear: vestibular labyrinth, cochlea	Superior cerebellum, including superior vermis, dentate nucleus
Core cerebellar syndrome	Isolated acute vestibular syndrome without auditory symptoms (pseudo-vestibular neuritis)	Isolated acute vestibular syndrome with auditory symptoms (pseudo-labyrinthitis)	Acute gait or trunk instability with associated dysarthria (pseudo-intoxication), nausea, or vomiting (pseudo-gastroenteritis)
Indicative neurologic signs	Lateral medullary syndrome: hemifacial analgesia, unilateral absent gag reflex, palatal palsy, vocal cord palsy, Horner syndrome, body hemianalgesia, limb hemiataxia, dysmetria	Lateral pontine syndrome: hemifacial sensory loss, facial palsy (lower motor neuron type), Horner syndrome, body hemianalgesia, limb hemiataxia, dysmetria	Lateral midbrain syndrome: fourth nerve palsy, hemifacial sensory loss, Horner syndrome, body hemisensory loss, limb hemiataxia, dysmetria
	Vertebral artery syndrome: 12th nerve palsy, body hemisensory loss, hemiplegia, or quadriplegia	Mid-basilar syndrome: impaired arousal or coma, sixth nerve palsy or internuclear ophthalmoplegia, horizontal gaze palsy, body hemisensory loss, hemiplegia, or quadriplegia	Top of the basilar syndrome: impaired memory or attention, visual field cut, ptosis, third nerve palsy, vertical gaze palsy, hemiplegia, or quadriplegia

deficits, and (4) a modest contraversive tilt of the subjective visual vertical (SVV) with otherwise normal vestibular function.[17]

Anterior inferior cerebellar artery infarction

Likewise in PICA infarction, vertigo is the common symptom of AICA territory infarction. However, AICA infarctions mostly accompany unilateral or bilateral hearing loss with or without brainstem signs such as facial palsy, Horner syndrome, or crossed sensory loss.[18] Direction-changing GEN similar to Bruns' nystagmus may be observed. Hearing loss is usually permanent, but dizziness and imbalance gradually improve with central compensation.

Because the AICA gives off the internal auditory artery that supplies the inner ear, AICA infarction typically causes combined peripheral and central vestibulopathy.[19] However, isolated labyrinthine infarction should be considered in older patients with sudden onset of unilateral deafness and vertigo, particularly if there is a history of stroke or known vascular risk factors. Because current imaging techniques cannot identify isolated labyrinthine infarction, the diagnosis should depend on clinical findings and concurrent vascular risk factors and remain presumptive without a pathologic study.[5]

The flocculus, also supplied by the AICA, is involved in the control of smooth tracking, gaze-holding, and eye movement induced by vestibular stimulation.[20] Previously, a patient with isolated unilateral floccular infarction showed spontaneous nystagmus beating to the lesion side, impaired ipsilesional pursuit, and contraversive ocular torsion and tilt of the SVV. With rotatory chair testing at low frequencies of stimulation, the horizontal vestibulo-ocular reflex (VOR) gains were increased. In contrast, the VOR gains were decreased with higher-frequency, higher-speed HITs.[20] Although the HITs are often normal in patients with central vestibular disorders, decreased HIT responses do not exclude an isolated cerebellar lesion involving the flocculus as a cause of AVS.

Superior cerebellar artery stroke

Because the superior cerebellum supplied by the SCA does not have significant vestibular connections, SCA territory infarction rarely causes vertigo. The low incidence of vertigo in SCA distribution may be useful for clinical distinction from PICA or AICA infarction in patients with acute unsteadiness. Lateral SCA infarction usually presents dizziness, unsteadiness, and mild truncal ataxia, but severe limb ataxia.[21] In contrast, the most prominent feature of medial SCA infarctions is severe gait ataxia with a sudden fall or severe veering.[21]

Medullary Infarction

Vertigo from brainstem strokes typically accompanies the symptoms and signs suggestive of a central lesion, thus constituting typical syndromes.

Lateral medullary infarction (Wallenberg syndrome)

As described in the introductory case, vertigo in lateral medullary infarction is usually associated with other neurologic symptoms or signs, including crossed sensory loss, Horner syndrome, limb ataxia, and ocular lateropulsion, causing little diagnostic challenge at the bedside.[5] However, tiny infarctions involving the lateral medulla may cause vertigo and unsteadiness without other localizing symptoms.[22] Spontaneous nystagmus in lateral medullary infarction varies considerably. Typically, the horizontal nystagmus beats away from the lesion side.[23] The vertical component is usually upbeating, but may be dissociated. The torsional nystagmus may be either ipsilesional or contralesional.[24] GEN is observed in almost all the patients, which is mostly horizontal. HSN is frequent, and the horizontal component of HSN is mostly ipsilesional.[23]

Even in patients with contralesional spontaneous nystagmus, horizontal HSN beat to the lesion side.[23] The ocular tilt reaction is an invariable finding during the acute phase and is ipsiversive, that is, the head is tilted to the lesion side, the upper poles of the eyes rotate toward the ipsilesional shoulder, and the ipsilesional eye lies lower than the contralesional one. Patients also show an oculomotor bias toward the lesion side without limitation of eye motion (ipsipulsion). The ocular ipsipulsion includes a steady-state ocular deviation to the lesion side, hypermetric ipsilesional saccades, and hypometric contralesional saccades opposite the lesion, and oblique misdirection of the vertical saccades.[23] Cervical and ocular vestibular-evoked myogenic potentials (VEMPs) also can be abnormal in Wallenberg syndrome.[25]

Medial medullary infarction

In medial medullary infarction, vertigo and oculomotor findings may be prominent when the lesions extend to the rostral tegmentum where the anteromedial arteries irrigate the ascending efferent fibers from the vestibular nuclei, medial longitudinal fasciculus (MLF), the perihypoglossal nuclear complex, the climbing fibers emanating from the inferior olive, and the cell groups of the paramedian tracts.[26] Medial medullary infarction generates distinct patterns of oculomotor abnormalities.[26] Spontaneous horizontal nystagmus usually beats to the lesion side.[26] GEN is usually more intense on looking ipsilesionally.[26] Upbeat or hemiseesaw nystagmus occasionally occurs and has been ascribed to the involvement of the perihypoglossal nuclei or MLF. Ocular contrapulsion may be observed owing to damage to the olivocerebellar fibers before decussation.[27] Damage to the medial vestibulospinal tract descending in the MLF may impair cervical VEMPs in the lesion side.[28]

Vestibular nuclear infarct

Infarctions restricted to the vestibular nuclei can cause isolated vertigo and nystagmus mimicking acute peripheral vestibulopathy.[29] The vestibular nuclei are supplied by both AICA and PICA. A recent analysis of patients with an isolated vestibular nucleus infarction described isolated prolonged vertigo, spontaneous horizontal-torsional nystagmus usually beating away from the lesion side, positive HITs, and unilateral caloric paresis.[29] Cervical and ocular VEMPs were decreased or absent during stimulation of the ipsilesional ear.[29] All of these findings are consistent with vestibular neuritis. However, the patients showed direction-changing GEN that is a typical sign of central vestibulopathy.[29] Isolated vestibular nucleus infarction should be considered in the differential diagnosis of AVS with features of combined peripheral and central vestibulopathy, especially when hearing is preserved.[19,29]

BEDSIDE AND LABORATORY DIAGNOSTIC TESTS

When other neurologic symptoms and signs are associated with acute dizziness/vertigo, the diagnosis of stroke is straightforward in most cases even without neuroimaging. However, acute vascular dizziness/vertigo with inconspicuous other neurologic deficits could escape detection even with MRIs and be challenging even for specialists. Recent progress in clinical neurotology, however, has proved that systematic bedside evaluation is superior to neuroimaging in diagnosing acute prolonged vertigo from strokes.[10,30]

Bedside Evaluation

Patients with acute prolonged vertigo should have an evaluation for spontaneous and provoked nystagmus; ocular misalignment, including skew deviation, saccades, and smooth pursuit in both horizontal and vertical directions; HITs; and balance function.[31]

Bedside HIT is a useful tool for differentiating central vascular vertigo syndrome from a more benign disorder involving the inner ear.[10,15] Normal HIT is a reliable sign for intact peripheral vestibular function, and is suggestive of a central lesion in patients with acute prolonged vertigo.[10,15,32] The diagnostic accuracy of a bedside HIT for differentiating central vascular vertigo from acute peripheral vestibulopathy may be enhanced if other central signs are combined. A refined bedside examination protocol that incorporated HIT, direction-changing nystagmus, and skew deviation (HINTS to INFARCT [Impulse Normal, Fast-phase Alternating or Refixation on Cover-Test]) showed a 100% sensitivity and 96% specificity in identifying strokes in patients with acute prolonged vertigo of more than 24 hours and one vascular risk factor, whereas initial diffusion-weighted MRIs were normal in 12%.[10] However, the HINTS may not be sufficiently robust to detect an AICA infarction because the HIT is mostly positive in this disorder. Indeed, the HINTS failed to detect central lesions in 5 of 18 patients with AICA infarction.[33] In those cases, addition of horizontal head shaking and hearing test with finger rub (HINTS plus) may aid in detecting a central lesion.[30,33]

Because a mild degree of skew deviation may go unnoticed during bedside examination and GEN is usually absent in cerebellar strokes, bedside HIT may be the best tool for differentiating isolated vertigo due to cerebellar strokes from acute peripheral vestibulopathy. However, bedside HIT may be false negative especially when the vestibular deficits are partial or the corrective saccades occur during the HIT (covert saccades).[34] In this respect, the recently developed video-based equipment for HIT would be helpful for objective measurements of head impulse VOR gains.[35,36]

Laboratory Tests

In general, routine laboratory studies, including complete blood counts, electrolytes, and thyroid function tests, have a very low yield in diagnosing a cause of dizziness. In a meta-analysis, only 26 (0.6%) of 4538 patients had laboratory abnormalities that could explain their dizziness.[37] The ischemic stroke guidelines also recommend a limited number of hematologic, coagulation, and biochemistry tests during the initial emergency evaluation, and only the assessment of blood glucose must precede the initiation of intravenous recombinant tissue plasminogen activator (rtPA).[38] Baseline electrocardiogram and troponin also are recommended in patients with acute ischemic stroke, but should not delay the initiation of intravenous rtPA.[38]

Neuroimaging studies are essential to confirm strokes. Computed tomography (CT) has a limited value in detecting posterior circulation infarction, and is recommended only to detect hemorrhages.[39] Even diffusion-weighted MRIs fail to disclose up to 1 in 5 strokes occurring in the posterior fossa during the first 24 to 48 hours.[11] Diffusion-weighted MRIs showed a lesser sensitivity than HINTS plus (HINTS plus bedside hearing by finger rub) in detecting small strokes (47% vs 100%, $P<.001$).[30] False-negative initial MRIs (6–48 hours) were more common with small strokes than larger ones (53% vs 7.8%, $P<.001$).[30] Thus, serial evaluation is required to confirm stroke in patients with suspected vascular vertigo when the initial diffusion MRIs were normal (**Fig. 3**).

Patients with suspected vascular vertigo should have a prompt assessment of cerebral vasculature using CT, magnetic resonance, or conventional angiography.[4,5] Perfusion imaging may help diagnose vascular vertigo, especially in patients with normal routine neuroimaging, and decide the extent of hypoperfusion.[40] However, the diagnostic yield of perfusion imaging should be validated in isolated vascular vertigo.

Various laboratory tests may be applied to evaluate vestibular and ocular motor function in patients with stroke, which is beyond the scope of this article.

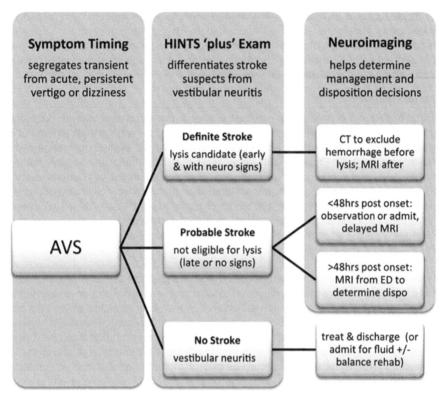

Fig. 3. Possible diagnostic strategy in AVS based on HINTS results. (*Adapted from* Jauch EC, Saver JL, Adams HP Jr, et al. Guidelines for the early management of patients with acute ischemic stroke: a guideline for healthcare professionals from the American Heart Association/American Stroke Association. Stroke 2013;44:870–947.)

ACUTE TREATMENT OPTIONS
General Principle

Because there have been no randomized trials that are specific for posterior circulation strokes, including cerebellar infarctions, the treatments for vascular vertigo should follow the guidelines for acute stroke in general.[39]

Wherever the patient is admitted, close monitoring of the signs of deterioration is crucial. If deterioration occurs, primary brainstem ischemia from the original vascular lesion must be distinguished from secondary brainstem compression or hydrocephalus because the treatment options for each differ. MRIs may help to make this distinction. Therefore, patients with acute cerebellar infarction should ideally be managed in a stroke center with a neurologic intensive care unit where close clinical monitoring, rapid access to brain imaging, and on-call neurosurgical expertise are readily available.[38]

Medical Treatments

Fluid and electrolyte imbalances should be monitored and corrected in patients with severe vomiting. Vestibular suppressants along with restriction in head motion may be applied to the patients with severe vertigo, nausea, and vomiting during the first few days. As soon as tolerated, the medication should be tapered, and vestibular rehabilitation should be initiated. According to the current guidelines,[38] isolated vascular vertigo is not indicated for thrombolysis due to its low disability score. However, prevention of future events should be attempted through strict control of the risk factors and use of antiplatelets or anticoagulation.

Surgical Treatments

Carotid endarterectomy/stenting may be beneficial in selected patients with dizziness/vertigo and concurrent vascular variants or anomaly, such as persistent trigeminal or persistent hypoglossal artery, which connects the carotid system to the posterior circulation directly.[41] Patients with large cerebellar infarctions are at high risk for complicating brain edema and increased intracranial pressure. Decompression should be considered in patients with deterioration due to direct brainstem compression or hydrocephalus. Placement of stents or surgery may be considered in patients with severe symptomatic vertebral artery stenosis, subclavian steal phenomenon, or rotational vertebral artery syndrome that is refractory to medical treatments.[42]

Rehabilitation

Stroke rehabilitation should be started as quickly as possible and can last anywhere from a few days to more than a year, even though most return of function is seen within the first few months. Vestibular rehabilitation is effective in reducing symptoms and improving function for patients with vestibular disorders. The goal of vestibular rehabilitation is to promote central nervous system compensation through exercise-based strategies. Thus, recovery may be limited in individuals with central vestibular dysfunction because involvement of the central vestibular structures can restrict compensation. The length of therapy is typically longer for those with central vestibular dysfunction.[43]

TRIAGE AND DISPOSITION

Within 4.5 hours of stroke (hyperacute phase), patients with AVS due to stroke should be considered for intravenous thrombolysis or acute endovascular surgery when the National Institutes of Health Stroke Scale (NIHSS) is greater than 4 or in cases with lower NIHSS that will clearly produce significant disability. Conservative treatments, including antiplatelet agents, strict risk factor management, and monitoring of deterioration may be sufficient for AVS in isolation or AVS associated with minimal disability such as internuclear ophthalmoplegia.

After 4.5 hours from stroke, AVS due to basilar artery occlusion may still be a candidate for intravenous thrombolysis or acute endovascular therapy. Otherwise, conservative management is the mainstay of the treatments. Patients with a completed stroke should be admitted because approximately 25% of patients may have neurologic worsening during the first 24 to 48 hours after stroke and it is difficult to predict which patients will deteriorate. Likewise, the patients with posterior circulation transient ischemic attack may have a benefit from admission for rapid assessment and close observation. Patients with deterioration from brain edema, hydrocephalus, and resultant compression of the brainstem should be taken promptly for decompressive surgery to limit secondary damage of previously noninfarcted portions of the brain.[38]

SUPPLEMENTARY DATA

Supplementary data related to this article can be found online at http://dx.doi.org/10.1016/j.ncl.2015.04.006.

REFERENCES

1. Kerber KA. Vertigo presentations in the emergency department. Semin Neurol 2009;29:482–90.
2. Fisher CM. Vertigo in cerebrovascular disease. Arch Otolaryngol 1967;85: 529–34.
3. Choi JH, Kim HW, Choi KD, et al. Isolated vestibular syndrome in posterior circulation stroke: frequency and involved structures. Neurol Clin Pract 2014;4:410–8.
4. Choi KD, Lee H, Kim JS. Vertigo in brainstem and cerebellar strokes. Curr Opin Neurol 2013;26:90–5.
5. Kim JS, Lee H. Vertigo due to posterior circulation stroke. Semin Neurol 2013;33: 179–84.
6. Kerber KA, Brown DL, Lisabeth LD, et al. Stroke among patients with dizziness, vertigo, and imbalance in the emergency department: a population-based study. Stroke 2006;37:2484–7.
7. Lee CC, Ho HC, Su YC, et al. Increased risk of vascular events in emergency room patients discharged home with diagnosis of dizziness or vertigo: a 3-year follow-up study. PLoS One 2012;7:e35923.
8. Lee CC, Su YC, Ho HC, et al. Risk of stroke in patients hospitalized for isolated vertigo: a four-year follow-up study. Stroke 2011;42:48–52.
9. Saber Tehrani AS, Coughlan D, Hsieh YH, et al. Rising annual costs of dizziness presentations to U.S. emergency departments. Acad Emerg Med 2013;20:689–96.
10. Kattah JC, Talkad AV, Wang DZ, et al. HINTS to diagnose stroke in the acute vestibular syndrome: three-step bedside oculomotor examination more sensitive than early MRI diffusion-weighted imaging. Stroke 2009;40:3504–10.
11. Tarnutzer AA, Berkowitz AL, Robinson KA, et al. Does my dizzy patient have a stroke? A systematic review of bedside diagnosis in acute vestibular syndrome. CMAJ 2011;183:E571–92.
12. Donnan GA, Fisher M, Macleod M, et al. Stroke. Lancet 2008;371:1612–23.
13. Lee H, Sohn SI, Cho YW, et al. Cerebellar infarction presenting isolated vertigo: frequency and vascular topographical patterns. Neurology 2006;67:1178–83.
14. Huh YE, Kim JS. Patterns of spontaneous and head-shaking nystagmus in cerebellar infarction: imaging correlations. Brain 2011;134:3662–71.
15. Newman-Toker DE, Kattah JC, Alvernia JE, et al. Normal head impulse test differentiates acute cerebellar strokes from vestibular neuritis. Neurology 2008;70: 2378–85.
16. Moon IS, Kim JS, Choi KD, et al. Isolated nodular infarction. Stroke 2009;40: 487–91.
17. Lee SH, Park SH, Kim JS, et al. Isolated unilateral infarction of the cerebellar tonsil: ocular motor findings. Ann Neurol 2014;75:429–34.
18. Lee H, Kim JS, Chung EJ, et al. Infarction in the territory of anterior inferior cerebellar artery: spectrum of audiovestibular loss. Stroke 2009;40:3745–51.
19. Choi SY, Kee HJ, Park JH, et al. Combined peripheral and central vestibulopathy. J Vestib Res 2014;24:443–51.
20. Park HK, Kim JS, Strupp M, et al. Isolated floccular infarction: impaired vestibular responses to horizontal head impulse. J Neurol 2013;260:1576–82.
21. Lee H. Neuro-otological aspects of cerebellar stroke syndrome. J Clin Neurol 2009;5:65–73.
22. Kim JS. Vertigo and gait ataxia without usual signs of lateral medullary infarction: a clinical variant related to rostral-dorsolateral lesions. Cerebrovasc Dis 2000;10: 471–4.

23. Choi KD, Oh SY, Park SH, et al. Head-shaking nystagmus in lateral medullary infarction: patterns and possible mechanisms. Neurology 2007;68:1337–44.

24. Morrow MJ, Sharpe JA. Torsional nystagmus in the lateral medullary syndrome. Ann Neurol 1988;24:390–8.

25. Oh SY, Kim JS, Lee JM, et al. Ocular vestibular evoked myogenic potentials induced by air-conducted sound in patients with acute brainstem lesions. Clin Neurophysiol 2013;124:770–8.

26. Kim JS, Choi KD, Oh SY, et al. Medial medullary infarction: abnormal ocular motor findings. Neurology 2005;65:1294–8.

27. Kim JS, Moon SY, Kim KY, et al. Ocular contrapulsion in rostral medial medullary infarction. Neurology 2004;63:1325–7.

28. Kim S, Lee HS, Kim JS. Medial vestibulospinal tract lesions impair sacculo-collic reflexes. J Neurol 2010;257:825–32.

29. Kim HJ, Lee SH, Park JH, et al. Isolated vestibular nuclear infarction: report of two cases and review of the literature. J Neurol 2014;261:121–9.

30. Saber Tehrani AS, Kattah JC, Mantokoudis G, et al. Small strokes causing severe vertigo: frequency of false-negative MRIs and nonlacunar mechanisms. Neurology 2014;83:169–73.

31. Huh YE, Kim JS. Bedside evaluation of dizzy patients. J Clin Neurol 2013;9: 203–13.

32. Newman-Toker DE, Kerber KA, Hsieh YH, et al. HINTS outperforms ABCD2 to screen for stroke in acute continuous vertigo and dizziness. Acad Emerg Med 2013;20:986–96.

33. Huh YE, Koo JW, Lee H, et al. Head-shaking aids in the diagnosis of acute audio-vestibular loss due to anterior inferior cerebellar artery infarction. Audiol Neurootol 2013;18:114–24.

34. MacDougall HG, Weber KP, McGarvie LA, et al. The video head impulse test: diagnostic accuracy in peripheral vestibulopathy. Neurology 2009;73:1134–41.

35. Newman-Toker DE, Saber Tehrani AS, Mantokoudis G, et al. Quantitative video-oculography to help diagnose stroke in acute vertigo and dizziness: toward an ECG for the eyes. Stroke 2013;44:1158–61.

36. Chen L, Todd M, Halmagyi GM, et al. Head impulse gain and saccade analysis in pontine-cerebellar stroke and vestibular neuritis. Neurology 2014;83:1513–22.

37. Hoffman RM, Einstadter D, Kroenke K. Evaluating dizziness. Am J Med 1999;107: 468–78.

38. Jauch EC, Saver JL, Adams HP Jr, et al. Guidelines for the early management of patients with acute ischemic stroke: a guideline for healthcare professionals from the American Heart Association/American Stroke Association. Stroke 2013;44: 870–947.

39. Edlow JA, Newman-Toker DE, Savitz SI. Diagnosis and initial management of cerebellar infarction. Lancet Neurol 2008;7:951–64.

40. Kim DU, Han MK, Kim JS. Isolated recurrent vertigo from stenotic posterior inferior cerebellar artery. Otol Neurotol 2011;32:180–2.

41. Zhou Y, Lee SH, Mantokoudis G, et al. Vertigo and dizziness in anterior circulation cerebrovascular disease: a systematic review. Neurology 2014;82(Suppl):3.092.

42. Kernan WN, Ovbiagele B, Black HR, et al. Guidelines for the prevention of stroke in patients with stroke and transient ischemic attack: a guideline for healthcare professionals from the American Heart Association/American Stroke Association. Stroke 2014;45:2160–236.

43. Whitney SL, Rossi MM. Efficacy of vestibular rehabilitation. Otolaryngol Clin North Am 2000;33:659–72.

Medical and Nonstroke Neurologic Causes of Acute, Continuous Vestibular Symptoms

Jonathan A. Edlow, MD[a],*, David E. Newman-Toker, MD, PhD[b]

KEYWORDS

• Acute vestibular syndrome • Neurologic disease • Dizziness • Stroke
• Multiple sclerosis

KEY POINTS

- Although isolated dizziness is an unusual presentation of multiple sclerosis (MS), in patients with the acute vestibular syndrome (AVS) who do not have a stroke or vestibular neuritis, MS is the most common cause.
- Occasional patients with cerebellar mass present with an AVS if there is bleeding into the tumor, an acute increase in perilesional edema, or simply the mass growing to a threshold beyond which the pressure in the posterior fossa increases rapidly.
- Cerebellitis, from either an infectious or an inflammatory cause, can present with an AVS.
- Mal de debarquement is obvious in most patients in the context of recent travel on boat (or sometimes air).
- Patients with prior posterior circulation stroke may have recrudescence (unmasking) of symptoms due to a new toxic, metabolic, or infectious condition.

INTRODUCTION

Dizziness has a broad differential diagnosis. In a report of nearly 10,000 patients from the National Hospital Ambulatory Medical Care Survey database who had dizziness as a reason for visit to a US emergency department, half had a medical (ie, nonvestibular and noncerebrovascular) cause for their dizziness.[1] These conditions included cardiovascular, respiratory, toxicologic, metabolic, psychiatric, and other causes. About 15% of these medical causes were a dangerous diagnosis, as defined by a prespecified list

[a] Department of Emergency Medicine Administrative Offices, West CC-2, Beth Israel Deaconess Medical Center, 1 Deaconess Place, Boston, MA 02215, USA; [b] Departments of Neurology, Otolaryngology, and Epidemiology, The Johns Hopkins University School of Medicine & Bloomberg School of Public Health, The Johns Hopkins Hospital, CRB-II, Room 2M-03 North, 1550 Orleans Street, Baltimore, MD 21231, USA
* Corresponding author.
E-mail address: jedlow@bidmc.harvard.edu

Neurol Clin 33 (2015) 699–716
http://dx.doi.org/10.1016/j.ncl.2015.04.002   neurologic.theclinics.com
0733-8619/15/$ – see front matter © 2015 Elsevier Inc. All rights reserved.

of conditions that had potentially bad outcomes and were treatable (eg, myocardial infarction or carbon monoxide poisoning).[1]

Distinguishing various timing and trigger categories of patients with dizziness helps to narrow down the differential diagnosis and focus on serious treatable causes. Many medical causes commonly present with episodic dizziness or vertigo (eg, cardiac arrhythmia, orthostatic hypotension, transient hypoglycemia), and these are presented in another article by Meurer and colleagues elsewhere in this issue and are not discussed further here. Other medical and nonstroke neurologic disorders instead present with acute, continuous symptoms that mimic the more common presentations of postconcussive dizziness, vestibular neuritis, and stroke. AVS is usually defined as the rapid onset of dizziness or vertigo, nausea or vomiting, head motion intolerance, gait instability, and often nystagmus lasting for at least 24 hours. Internists, general practitioners, and especially emergency physicians frequently encounter a broader array of disorders causing AVS, such as toxic or metabolic disorders, infections, and inflammatory diseases. These disorders are the subject of this article.

Although most cases of definite AVS are likely to be either vestibular neuritis or stroke,[2] the differential diagnosis of the syndrome is broad (**Box 1**). Cases of AVS that are not posttraumatic, unilateral peripheral vestibulopathies (vestibular neuritis/labyrinthitis) or are with a cerebrovascular cause can be categorized into 3 general groups. The first group includes patients with general medical problems that are principally toxicologic, metabolic, or infectious (eg, a patient with phenytoin toxicity or hyponatremia). The second group includes neurologic conditions other than stroke (eg, MS, brainstem encephalitis). The third group includes patients with hybrid medical and neurologic causes in which subclinical neurologic or vestibular conditions (either in recovery or early in the disease state) are unmasked by intercurrent medical illness, causing acute symptoms.

Before discussion of these 3 groups of conditions, one additional caveat must be discussed. Some patients with a spontaneous episodic vestibular syndrome present before the episode resolves (eg, 4 hours after symptoms begin). Therefore, one cannot always readily distinguish these patients (in whom future spontaneous resolution would clarify the episodic nature of the process) from patients who will remain dizzy and therefore qualify as a true AVS case. Typical examples include patients with Meniere disease, vestibular migraine, or transient ischemic attack who present early, while still symptomatic. Just as a patient with transient ischemic attack should be treated presumptively as a patient with stroke if they remain symptomatic at clinical presentation, so too should these episodic patients be treated as an AVS case until subsequent events clarify the true nature of the event. Although they enter into differential diagnostic consideration, these conditions are discussed fully in other articles. Finally, dizziness in adults has been emphasized, recognizing that much less is known about AVS among children, other than a suspicion that strokes are less common and some disorders of childhood are likely to be more common (eg, genetic disorders, cerebellitis, posterior fossa tumors).

GENERAL MEDICAL CONDITIONS WITHOUT OBVIOUS STRUCTURAL NEUROLOGIC DISEASE

Numerous toxicologic, metabolic, and systemic infectious conditions can cause some degree of persistent dizziness, although the proportion of such patients presenting with symptoms truly consistent with or closely mimicking an AVS, in the absence of other symptoms indicating a clear cause, is unknown. Experience would suggest

Box 1
Differential diagnosis of AVS

Benign[a] or Less Urgent Causes

  Common causes (>1% of AVS)

- Vestibular neuritis
- Multiple sclerosis

  Uncommon (<1%) or unknown frequency

- Viral labyrinthitis
- Herpes zoster oticus (Ramsay Hunt syndrome)
- Acute traumatic vestibulopathy
- Medication ototoxicity (eg, aminoglycosides)
- Acute disseminated encephalomyelitis
- CNS side effects (eg, antiepileptics)
- Prolonged Meniere syndrome attack
- Prolonged vestibular migraine attack
- Episodic ataxia syndrome attack
- Cerebellopontine angle neoplasm (eg, vestibular schwannoma, metastases)

  Presumed possible causes[c]

- Atypical infection (otosyphilis, Lyme disease)
- Degenerative cerebellar ataxia
- Drug intoxication (eg, alcohol, illicit substances)

Dangerous[a] and More Urgent Causes

  Common causes (>1% of AVS)

- Brainstem or cerebellar infarction
- Brainstem or cerebellar hemorrhage

  Uncommon (<1%) or unknown frequency

- Labyrinthine stroke[b]
- Bacterial labyrinthitis/mastoiditis
- Autoimmune vestibulopathy (eg, Cogan syndrome)
- Wernicke syndrome (B_1 deficiency)
- Miller Fisher syndrome
- Brainstem encephalitis or cerebellitis (eg, *Listeria*, herpes simplex/zoster, paraneoplastic, Creutzfeldt-Jakob disease)

  Presumed possible causes[c]

- Cerebral infarction or hemorrhage
- Subarachnoid hemorrhage/aneurysm
- Severe anemia or hypoxia
- Carbon monoxide toxicity
- Electrolyte (eg, hyponatremia, hyperglycemia)
- Endocrine (eg, hypothyroidism)
- Decompression sickness
- Mountain sickness
- Hypertensive encephalopathy
- CNS medication toxicity (eg, lithium)
- Ciguatera poisoning

Abbreviation: CNS, central nervous system.

[a] Any disease causing dizziness/vertigo can be considered a dangerous medical problem if the symptoms occur in dangerous circumstances (eg, highway driving or free-rock climbing). Furthermore, the high vagal tone that accompanies some vestibular disorders can provoke bradyarrhythmias in susceptible individuals, including during the examination.[111] Nevertheless, although they may be quite disabling to patients during the acute illness phase, diseases classified here as Benign or Less Urgent Causes rarely produce severe, irreversible morbidity or mortality (unlike their dangerous counterparts).

[b] The frequency of labyrinthine infarction is difficult to estimate given that the current reference standard test for confirming the diagnosis (ie, autopsy with temporal bone histology) is rarely performed. Recent studies, however, suggest that patients with sudden deafness, with or without vertigo, are at increased risk of stroke, suggesting a possible vascular mechanism.[112]

[c] Presumed possible causes are conditions known to cause acute dizziness, but it remains unknown whether they can present with a clinically complete or clinically predominant AVS picture.

Modified from Tarnutzer AA, Berkowitz AL, Robinson KA, et al. Does my dizzy patient have a stroke? A systematic review of bedside diagnosis in acute vestibular syndrome. CMAJ 2011;183:E571–92.

that the figure is low. In some such patients, a plausible pathophysiologic explanation (eg, anemia, fever, hypoxia, or cellular dysfunction due to presence of toxins and altered acid-base or electrolyte levels) exists. In others, the mechanism for dizziness remains unclear.

Pharmacologic Toxicity and Withdrawal

The most common medical causes of acute, continuous dizziness are pharmacologic intoxications. Clinically relevant examples of mechanistically distinct toxicities are provided later in the discussion. Intoxicants include both licit and illicit substances affecting the brainstem, cerebellum, or peripheral vestibular apparatus. Pharmacotherapies may cause acute dizziness as a side effect of treatment or, occasionally, treatment withdrawal.[3] Most patients experience a single, acute attack resolving gradually over days to weeks once the exposure to toxin has stopped. Depending on the nature of the toxin, other symptoms such as altered mental status may predominate. Rotatory vertigo, spontaneous nystagmus, and head motion intolerance (typical with vestibular neuritis and stroke) are more likely with unilateral dysfunction (eg, with phosphodiesterase inhibitors for erectile dysfunction, reported to cause unilateral hearing loss and vertigo, suggesting inner ear ischemia).[4] More often, however, these clinical features are absent, especially when a systemic toxin affects the peripheral vestibular apparatus in a symmetric manner. If an exposure is prolonged or severe, permanent damage may ensue and patients may transition directly into a chronic dizziness phase (eg, following severe aminoglycoside ototoxicity).[5]

Reversible acute dizziness or vertigo due to medication side effects or toxicity from overdosage is typical with central nervous system (CNS)-acting agents that have a brainstem or cerebellar predilection, such as antiepileptic drugs (especially phenytoin, carbamazepine, and phenobarbital), benzodiazepines, and lithium.[6] Anticonvulsants are perhaps most likely to mimic a true AVS presentation with severe persistent vertigo, dizziness, or ataxia in combination with pathologic nystagmus,[7,8] although similar presentations have also been reported for other medications, such as amiodarone.[9]

Acute alcohol intoxication produces dizziness by both central and peripheral mechanisms.[6,10] The resultant nystagmus can therefore be of a mixed type but is most commonly a direction-changing, gaze-evoked horizontal nystagmus (ie, beats to the right when looking right, beats to the left when looking left), as with other brainstem and cerebellar intoxicants, that results from impairment of central gaze-holding pathways. Alcohol use can also cause dizziness via other mechanisms such as thiamine deficiency (discussed later) and chronic cerebellar degeneration, although the last two mechanisms generally lead to a more chronic presentation, unless there is intercurrent medical illness.

Aminoglycoside toxicity to vestibular hair cells is a well-known cause of acute bilateral vestibular failure.[11,12] Gentamicin, the most commonly used modern agent, can produce profound, permanent loss of peripheral vestibular function with spared hearing, and toxicity may occur after even a single antibiotic dose.[11] Longer duration of therapy may increase the risk. Patients may experience an acute, severe unsteadiness with head motion intolerance followed by oscillopsia. Although this problem is usually discovered during the course of an inpatient hospital admission, patients may develop symptoms later and present to acute care. Early bedside detection might prove beneficial for some patients if the treatment can be stopped immediately.

Alcohol or opiate withdrawal can cause persistent dizziness symptoms, although presumably autonomic symptoms and signs usually make the cause fairly obvious. A withdrawal syndrome more likely to present with continuous dizziness without obvious features is that following discontinuation of selective serotonin reuptake inhibitors.[13] Symptoms generally peak within 3 to 5 days after stopping the medication and can last for weeks, and dizziness is the most common symptom.[13] Nystagmus may even be seen.[14] It has been postulated that this phenomenon results from acute serotonin depletion in the vestibular nuclear complex in the brainstem.[15] Typically, however, patients who develop this syndrome have less fulminant symptoms than a patient presenting AVS due to vestibular neuritis or stroke.

Environmental Toxins

There are numerous industrial chemicals that can cause dizziness; a complete list is beyond the scope of this article. Two well-known examples are volatile hydrocarbons (eg, acute toluene toxicity)[16] and pesticides (eg, pyrethroids and organophosphates).[17] Many environmental toxins prominently cause dizziness and typically also more specific symptoms (eg, muscarinic effects in organophosphate toxicity, such as salivation, lacrimation, and urination). Biotoxins may also cause acute dizziness or vertigo. A well-established and potentially lethal example is ciguatera, a form of fish poisoning endemic to certain tropical islands; the disorder is frequently characterized by the development of acute vertigo and ataxia, in addition to circumoral paresthesias.[18]

One toxin that may present with dizziness and headache on exposure, without more specific symptoms as a clue to the underlying cause, is carbon monoxide. The estimated prevalence of occult carbon monoxide exposure in patients presenting to an urban emergency department in the winter months with dizziness or headache was 3% to 5% in one study.[19] Because nausea and vomiting are frequent accompaniments,[20] the clinical features may closely mimic a more typical cause of AVS, especially in cases in which nystagmus is present.[21]

Electrolyte, Endocrine, and Micronutrient Disturbances

Fluid, electrolyte, and related abnormalities are commonly diagnosed in patients with dizziness who come to the emergency department, with these disorders diagnosed in 7% (5.6% fluid and electrolyte, 1.4% hypoglycemia) of a nationally representative sample of patients.[1] Most of these patients likely present with episodic dizziness symptoms, either due to volume depletion with orthostatic hypotension or due to transient hypoglycemia. However, some probably present with symptoms of persistent, nonepisodic dizziness or vertigo. It is unknown how often electrolyte (and related metabolic) disorders closely mimic vestibular neuritis or stroke presentations, and it is presumed that in most such cases nystagmus is absent, although, to the authors' knowledge, this has not been well studied. Although these are dangerous disorders that require prompt diagnosis and treatment, the typical care process in the emergency department (which involves routine laboratory tests for electrolytes and glucose in almost all patients presenting with dizziness) makes it highly unlikely that these disorders are frequently misdiagnosed in this care setting.

Alterations in blood glucose levels are the metabolic disturbances that are probably the most tightly linked to vestibular symptoms. Hypoglycemia, in particular, is a well-recognized cause of dizziness, and even vertigo.[22] In controlled intervention studies, transient induced hypoglycemia less than 5.6 mmol/L is associated with increased symptoms of dizziness.[23] Clinically, transient hypoglycemia, often due to overdosage of insulin or oral hypoglycemic agents, generally leads to temporary symptoms of dizziness, light-headedness, or unsteadiness, often accompanied by sweating, tremulousness, generalized weakness, and mental confusion.[24] However, because prolonged, severe hypoglycemia leads fairly rapidly to obtundation and coma, it is unusual for hypoglycemia to present with persistent dizziness per se.[25] Some studies suggest that hyperglycemia can also be associated with dizziness.[26] However, controlled experiments with transient induced hyperglycemia did not find an increase in dizziness symptoms up to a serum glucose level of 21 mmol/L.[23] Persistent stroke-like symptoms, seizures, and altered sensorium are well described in patients with severe hyperglycemic hyperosmolar syndrome, although vestibular disturbances (eg, nystagmus) are infrequently mentioned, perhaps because cerebral hemispheric, rather than brainstem, involvement predominates.[27] Thus, although theoretically possible, hyperglycemia is probably rarely a cause of persistent dizziness mimicking vestibular neuritis or stroke.

The most common electrolyte abnormality likely to present with persistent dizziness is almost certainly hyponatremia. Typical presentations involve a combination of dizziness, nausea, and vomiting,[28] so this clinical presentation might initially be confused for AVS due to stroke or inner ear disease. Care should be taken when correcting severe hyponatremia, because of the risk of inducing an osmotic demyelination syndrome.[29] Hypernatremia is more likely to cause dizziness via dehydration and orthostatic hypotension,[30] as the typical CNS symptoms of hyperosmolality are those of altered mental status, lethargy, irritability, restlessness, seizures, muscle twitching, hyperreflexia, and spasticity alongside fever, nausea or vomiting, labored respiration, and intense thirst.[31] Hypokalemia or hyperkalemia are also more likely to cause dizziness via bradycardia resulting in hypotensive effects.[32,33] Dizziness and vertigo have been reported as symptomatic manifestations of hypocalcemia, hypercalcemia, hypophosphatemia, hyperphosphatemia, and hypomagnesemia,[34–38] although mixed electrolyte disturbances or comorbid diseases (eg, renal failure, thyroid dysfunction) sometimes cloud inferences about causal relationships.

Endocrine disorders may manifest with dizziness, generally as part of a larger clinical syndrome. For some disorders, this is most often due to orthostatic hypotension (eg, adrenal insufficiency, diabetes insipidus), and the dizziness is therefore more likely to be transient and postural. In other cases, the proximate cause of the dizziness seems to be more direct and the symptoms may be more continuous. For example, patients with severe hypothyroidism (myxedema) may complain of persistent dizziness,[39,40] and those with acute hyperthyroidism (thyrotoxicosis/thyroid storm) may present with dizziness and tremor[41] or dizziness and severe vomiting.[42] There is some evidence that thyroid dysfunction causes a mix of peripheral vestibular[43] and cerebellar[40] effects. Although the mechanistic understanding of these effects remains limited, thyroid disorders may be more common than previously imagined in patients presenting with acute dizziness to the emergency department.[36]

Disorders of micronutrients can also be associated with dizziness or vertigo. Depletion of vitamin B_{12} or E may cause a cerebellar ataxia syndrome that is usually chronic and slowly progressive, but it may occasionally present over a few months or even a few weeks.[44,45] More likely to present acutely, however, is thiamine (vitamin B_1) deficiency. Wernicke syndrome is classically associated with malnourished alcoholic patients, but in the modern era, this entity actually occurs more frequently in patients with cancer, hyperemesis gravidarum, and restrictive dieting or after bariatric surgery.[46] The classic triad of eye signs, cerebellar dysfunction, and confusion is found only in 8% of patients.[46] Early symptoms are often related to balance dysfunction, and patients typically present with gait unsteadiness or ataxia. Patients with a dominantly vestibular presentation mimicking vestibular neuritis have also been reported.[47] The vast majority of patients with thiamine-deficient ataxia have bilateral, direction-changing, gaze-evoked nystagmus, but many also have impaired vestibular reflexes. It is now suspected that the combination of bilateral loss of vestibulo-ocular reflex function by head impulse testing together with bilateral gaze-evoked nystagmus may be almost pathognomonic in the correct clinical setting.[47] Furthermore, quantitative recordings have shown rapid reversal over a few days in vestibular deficits following intravenous thiamine administration.[47] Any patient presenting with dizziness or vertigo in the context of a known prior gastric bypass, intestinal malabsorption syndrome, or other reason for nutritional deficiency should be assessed promptly for vitamin deficiencies. Those likely to have thiamine deficiency should have no glucose administered, thiamine level determined, and intravenous thiamine administered promptly on presentation.

Cardiovascular, Respiratory, Rheological, and Hematologic Disturbances

Numerous disorders of cardiovascular function that lead to drops in blood pressure can present with dizziness or vertigo.[48] However, it is highly unusual for a condition to produce stable, sustained hypotension (low enough to be symptomatic without losing consciousness), present both lying and standing, that lasts days to weeks. Autonomic disorders such as postural orthostatic tachycardia syndrome frequently present with dizziness or vertigo, but the symptoms are almost invariably postural, dissipating entirely when the patient lies down. Early in the disease course, patients with dangerous diseases such as aortic dissection, myocardial infarction, pulmonary embolus, anaphylaxis, incipient sepsis, or catastrophic internal bleeding may have stable hypotension. If such patients are seen in the emergency department in the first few hours, they might initially be mistaken for an early AVS presentation because of vestibular neuritis, but nystagmus and head motion intolerance are typically absent. Hypertension is discussed later in the section on nonstroke CNS causes.

Unlike patients with hypotension, those who are hypoxic or anemic often have persistent and continuous dizziness or vertigo. The symptoms may be exacerbated by positional change or head movement, as in anemia,[49] but this is no different than vestibular neuritis or stroke presenting AVS. In many cases, particularly with hypoxia, the patient has confusion or altered mental status. The frequency with which such patients closely mimic typical AVS (eg, isolated vertigo, ataxia, nystagmus) is unknown. Regardless, given typical US emergency department practice, it would be rare to miss dizziness due to hypoxia, severe anemia, or other hematologic disorder, because every patient typically has both pulse oximetry done and complete blood count taken.

Unusual hematologic disorders associated with hyperviscosity or microangiopathy including plasma cell dyscrasias, polycythemia vera, essential thrombocytosis, intravascular lymphoma, leukemia, sickle cell anemia, thrombotic thrombocytopenic purpura, hemolytic uremic syndrome, and disseminated intravascular coagulation may present with neurologic symptoms, including dizziness or vertigo.[50–56] Vestibular effects may be due to vascular sludging or microinfarcts in either the vestibular periphery or CNS, but symptoms can occur without strokes evident by neuroimaging. Because these disorders can damage the vestibular end organ or CNS in a manner similar to more typical strokes, they could present as with AVS patients with vestibular neuritis or stroke. Nevertheless, abnormalities in routine laboratory tests are evident in most of these patients.

Two specific syndromes associated with small vascular occlusions whereby hematologic parameters are normal and patients often present for acute care to the emergency department deserve special mention here: decompression sickness (generally after recreational diving) and fat emboli syndrome (as seen following long bone fractures or after hip replacement surgery). Both conditions can present with dizziness or vertigo from ear or brain involvement, and imaging studies may be unremarkable. Inner ear decompression syndrome is the clinical variant most likely to mimic vestibular neuritis and should be considered even when divers present with isolated vertigo without hearing loss.[57]

NONSTROKE NEUROLOGIC CONDITIONS

There are probably hundreds of different nonstroke neurologic conditions that might be associated with dizziness or vertigo. Any disorders that have a particular predilection for the brainstem or cerebellum are most likely to present with vestibular symptoms. Four illness groups that often present this way deserve special mention here: demyelinating disease, posterior-fossa neoplasms, brainstem or cerebellar encephalitis, and disorders of intracranial pressure (ICP). Each is discussed, in turn, recognizing that a thorough treatment of these subjects is beyond the scope of this article.

Demyelinating Disease, Especially Multiple Sclerosis

Demyelinating diseases include MS, neuromyelitis optica, acute disseminated encephalomyelitis, and osmotic demyelination syndromes (as with pontine myelinolysis from rapid correction of hyponatremia). Of these, MS is the most common and the syndrome most likely to affect the brainstem and cerebellum, although posterior fossa involvement can occur in any demyelinating disease.

Dizziness is a common symptom in patients with MS, occurring in up to one-third of patients.[58] The frequency of AVS presentations of MS differs depending on whether the denominator is all patients with AVS or all patients with MS. In a prospective study of patients presenting with AVS, 7 of 170 (4%) were found to have MS as a cause, usually with active demyelinating lesions located in the brainstem or cerebellum.[59] Among the those cases of the AVS that have a central cause, a systematic review found only 14 or 126 (11%) were due to MS.[2] Studying this issue from the other direction, analysis of patients with MS, suggests that dizziness as an isolated symptom is probably an uncommon presentation of MS. In one study of 75 patients with a clinically isolated MS-like syndrome specifically involving the brainstem or cerebellum, diplopia (68%) was the most common symptom, not vertigo (19%) or unsteady gait (31%).[60] In a series of 483 patients with MS, isolated cranial nerve root involvement at initial clinical presentation occurred only in 7% of cases, and the eighth nerve was the least commonly involved.[61]

Finally, in patients with known MS who become dizzy, other causes of dizziness may be more common than an MS flare. In one large series of 1153 patients with MS, 78 (6.8%) developed dizziness at some point in time. Of the 25 patients who could be evaluated during the dizzy episode, 52% had benign paroxysmal positional vertigo as a cause, whereas only 32% had a new MS plaque as a cause.[62] Other specific causes included Meniere disease, vestibular neuritis, and vestibular migraine.

Posterior Fossa Neoplasms and Other Mass Lesions

Cerebellar mass lesions include benign and malignant primary CNS tumors and metastatic lesions, infectious conditions such as abscess, and vascular lesions (arteriovenous malformations [AVMs]). These lesions tend to grow slowly, so most patients with cerebellar masses present with a chronic vestibular syndrome due to gradual displacement of adjacent structures or destruction of cerebellar tissue. Common symptoms include a sense of unsteadiness with an ataxic or staggering gait and often clumsiness or ataxia of the limbs.[63] If acute obstructive hydrocephalus supervenes, the clinical picture shifts to one of headache, vomiting, and progressive deterioration of mental status. Nevertheless, some patients with cerebellar mass lesions present with acute ataxia and an AVS, although the frequency is unknown.[64] In one large emergency department–based study of 2671 patients with acute isolated vertigo, posterior fossa tumors were identified in 40 patients (1.5% of the total and 33% of those ultimately diagnosed with central causes); however, only 626 underwent MRI, so the study was potentially limited by incomplete diagnostic ascertainment.[65]

An AVS presentation can occur for 1 of 3 mechanistic reasons. First, a hemorrhage may occur within a neoplasm. Second, edema may develop adjacent to a posterior fossa neoplasm or abscess. Third, even a slow-growing mass will eventually reach a threshold volume such that the local posterior fossa pressure begins to increase quickly. The common pathophysiology of these 3 situations is that a small incremental change in the volume of the mass within the rigid confines of the posterior fossa has reached an inflection point, causing a rapid elevation in posterior fossa ICP. This condition accounts for the acute presentation and simultaneously creates urgency to timely diagnosis and intervention, often consisting of surgical decompression.

In children, posterior fossa neoplasms are more common than hemispheric brain tumors, including pilocytic astrocytomas, medulloblastomas, and ependymomas. In adults, the most common primary cerebellar and cerebellopontine tumors are vestibular schwannomas, meningiomas, hemangioblastomas, and lymphomas. Although glioblastoma is the most common primary brain tumor in adults, primary glioblastoma in the cerebellum is rare.[66,67] Rarely, an unruptured AVM or aneurysm can present as AVS by compression or displacement of adjacent tissue.[63] Abscesses can also present as mass lesions, and these are described in the next section.

One specific management decision arises in patients with a new symptomatic presentation of a suspected posterior fossa neoplasm. Clinicians must decide whether or not to administer intravenous steroids to reduce edema. With the caveat that patients who are rapidly deteriorating should be treated, it is important to remember that even a single dose of steroid can render the histology of a biopsy specimen uninterpretable in patients with CNS lymphoma.[68,69] Because this can negatively affect subsequent management decisions, early coordination with an oncologist and/or neurosurgeon is important. In some cases, decompressive biopsy (and not empiric steroids) may be the best first step.

Many patients with metastatic disease have a history of a known cancer; however, just as for any cancer, in some patients, a metastasis can be the presenting symptom. In one series of patients, a cerebellar metastasis caused the presenting symptoms in 25% of cases (15 of 59).[70] Therefore, even in a patient without a known history of a systemic cancer, a new cerebellar mass could be due to a metastasis. Analysis of registry data suggests that cerebellar location of brain metastases is increasing.[71] The most common primary tumor site is the lung, with the breast, melanoma, and colon making up a large proportion of the rest.[70] Headache is more common than dizziness, but the 2 symptoms often co-occur. Because headache is uncommon in vestibular neuritis, co-occurrence of headache and dizziness in AVS usually suggests a central cause such as stroke or mass lesion.

Brainstem/Cerebellar Encephalitis (Infectious and Autoimmune Conditions)

Brainstem and cerebellar inflammation, sometimes called rhombencephalitis, can be caused by an infectious or noninfectious/parainfectious autoimmune process. Available case series tend to lump together patients with many different underlying causes. These causes include infections (eg, Listeria, herpes simplex) and other autoimmune conditions (eg, Miller Fisher syndrome and paraneoplastic encephalitis).

With infectious causes, isolated AVS presentations are generally uncommon; headache, fever, and altered mental status are often prominent symptoms. However, in cerebellar brain abscess, the possibility exists that a patient could present with an isolated AVS. Only a minority of patients with brain abscess has the diagnostic triad of fever, headache, and altered level of consciousness.[72] Empirically, dizziness is a rare presenting symptom for brain abscess.[72,73] However, when the diagnosis is under consideration, lumbar puncture (LP) should be avoided, because the cerebrospinal fluid (CSF) only yields the causative organism in approximately 25% of cases and because LP can be life threatening, especially in patients with posterior fossa abscess or subdural empyema.[72,74] Depending on the epidemiologic context, a variety of unusual organisms must be considered, including *Mycobacterium tuberculosis*, *Treponema pallidum*, *Toxoplasma gondii*, *Taenia soleum*, and various fungal species.[74,75]

Infectious encephalitis, in contrast to abscesses, nearly always presents with some combination of fever, headache, or altered mental status, and, with cerebral hemispheric involvement, often seizures. In one large series, dizziness was not listed as a presenting symptom,[76] but this was not a series focused specifically on rhombencephalitis cases. Vertigo and dizziness, therefore, are not usually symptoms of typical encephalitis.

Among cases of infectious rhombencephalitis, *Listeria* is the most common cause.[77] The disease disproportionately affects healthy young adults. It typically presents with a biphasic course that begins as a flulike syndrome followed by brainstem and cerebellar dysfunction, whereby vertigo and ataxia are common features.[78] This clinical presentation can easily be mistaken for vestibular neuritis after a viral syndrome[79] with potentially devastating consequences for patients, because early treatment is critical. In the preantibiotic era, mortality was 66%, compared with 20% to –30% in the antibiotic era.[78] Diagnosis is generally made by repeated CSF or blood cultures; the laboratory should be notified of the clinical suspicion, because the organisms are fastidious and cultures are falsely negative in roughly half of cases.[78] Optimal treatment is with ampicillin, and it is critical to note that typical empiric meningitis treatments with third-generation cephalosporins are ineffective. Rhombencephalitis may also be caused by enteroviruses (especially enterovirus 71), flaviviruses (especially Japanese encephalitis virus), and herpesviruses (especially herpes simplex virus). Both herpes simplex and herpes zoster viral infections have been reported to begin as more typical vestibular neuritis or Ramsay Hunt syndrome and progress to frank encephalitis.[80,81] Other atypical bacterial infections are rare causes, including tuberculosis, brucellosis, legionella, and mycoplasma infections.[78] In cases with relevant travel or environmental exposures, these other disorders should be considered.

Noninfectious rhombencephalitis includes the autoimmune, postinfectious Miller Fisher syndrome and the related disorder Bickerstaff encephalitis. Classic Miller Fisher syndrome presents with the triad of ataxia, ophthalmoplegia, and areflexia and is generally considered a variant of Guillain-Barré syndrome. Most cases are seen after an infection (typically a mild diarrheal illness due to *Campylobacter jejuni*) and have circulating anti-Gq1b antibodies, elevated levels of CSF protein without increased cell counts (albuminocytologic dissociation), and generally normal results on neuroimaging.[64,82] More than half of those with so-called Bickerstaff encephalitis have additional brainstem features at presentation such as limb weakness or diplopia and go on to have altered level of consciousness later in the illness.[83] Some initially present with dizziness or vertigo, although subacute ataxia is a more common presentation. More typical cases of Guillain-Barré syndrome may also present with an ataxic disturbance due to severe sensory loss. Regardless of the specific disorder, careful early monitoring of the patient's ventilatory status is critical because early complications are mainly due to respiratory failure.

Even in acute cerebellitis (ie, without direct brainstem involvement), whereby one might imagine a pure vestibular presentation was the rule rather than the exception, isolated ataxia is surprisingly uncommon.[84] Instead, headaches, vomiting, and lethargy, with or without fever, dominate the clinical descriptions of most cases (among 18 cases, none presented with isolated AVS).[85] Nevertheless, AVS presentations closely mimicking vestibular neuritis or stroke do occasionally occur, as in the case of an adult patient who presented with acute dizziness and was diagnosed as acute cerebellitis by both CSF analysis and MRI.[86] Causes for acute cerebellitis include a variety of viral (eg, herpes zoster or Epstein-Barr virus) or atypical bacterial infections,[82] and even Creutzfeldt-Jakob disease,[87] but most cases remain of unknown cause and are presumed to be autoimmune.[85]

Some of these autoimmune cases in adults represent paraneoplastic cerebellopathy syndromes linked to a known or, more often, occult malignancy. The immune response to the neoplasm often controls malignant proliferation but leads to collateral damage to neurons, presumably through immunologic cross-reactivity. Typical neoplasms include testicular, breast, ovarian, small-cell lung, and lymphoma. Sometimes circulating autoantibodies may be found in paraneoplastic cerebellitis (particularly anti-Yo, anti-Ri, anti-Tr) or brainstem encephalitis (particularly anti-Hu, anti-Ma2, anti-CRMP5).[88] The most effective treatment is to find and remove the underlying tumor—time is of the essence, because progressive neurologic deterioration is often nonreversible. On occasion, symptoms closely mimic a typical AVS presentation.[89]

Typical bacterial pathogens can spread from the middle ear (otitis media) initially to the labyrinth, leading to AVS symptoms, but ultimately progressing to potentially lethal meningitis or dural venous sinus thrombosis.[89,90] Otoscopy is essential in any AVS presentation to rule out otitis media and cholesteatoma, particularly in patients with otorrhea or a history of middle ear surgery. More than half of bacterial labyrinthitis cases with AVS presentations and nystagmus have an irritative rather than destructive pattern, with the nystagmus beating toward the diseased ear.[91]

Lyme disease and syphilis can affect the vestibular system and CNS but rarely do so in fulminant fashion. Both Lyme disease and syphilis are occasional causes of vestibular neuritis presenting an AVS clinical picture.[92,93] Rare autoimmune (eg, sarcoidosis, Behçet disease, Cogan syndrome, Vogt-Koyanagi-Harada syndrome) or vasculopathic (eg, Susac syndrome) diseases with a special predilection for inner ear and ocular involvement can also mimic vestibular neuritis.

Disorders of Intracranial Pressure and Brain Edema

Patients with elevated ICP, including that due to idiopathic intracranial hypertension (pseudotumor cerebri), may present with vertigo or dizziness, typically in association with pulsatile tinnitus, although headache is far more likely to be the chief symptom. In the emergency department, atypical features are common, and papilledema may be absent[94] or difficult to detect.[95] Patients with dural venous sinus thrombosis may present similarly[96] and are at risk for progression and neurologic deterioration.[97]

Other disorders associated with elevated ICP include obstructive or communicating hydrocephalus. Communicating hydrocephalus may be secondary to cryptococcal meningitis, which often presents with headaches and unsteady gait; it can also present with AVS mimicking vestibular neuritis.[98]

Brain edema occurs in a family of related disorders that includes posterior reversible encephalopathy syndrome, hypertensive encephalopathy, and eclampsia.[99,100] Acute mountain sickness presents with headaches, vomiting, and dizziness, with prevalence increasing from just more than 10% at 3000 m to just more than 50% at 4500 m above sea level.[101] In its most severe form, it is associated with high-altitude cerebral edema, with some features similar to hypertensive encephalopathy. These are dominantly cerebral hemispheric syndromes, but similar disorders can affect the brainstem and have been called reversible brainstem hypertensive encephalopathy.[102] Although dizziness is frequently attributed to hypertension in the emergency department, the causal link in patients without hypertensive encephalopathy is not firmly established. For example, although headaches and dizziness were both found to be common in adults presenting to the emergency department with hypertensive crisis, they were equally common in a control group with uncomplicated hypertension.[103] In children, there may be a stronger association between hypertensive crisis and dizziness.[104]

Patients with intracranial hypotension following LP or spontaneous CSF leak may also present with auditory or vestibular symptoms, including acute vertigo.[105]

PHYSIOLOGIC UNMASKING OF OCCULT OR RECOVERED NEUROLOGIC DISEASE

Many patients have chronic neurologic conditions that affect balance and vestibular function that are sufficiently compensated so that under normal circumstances they do not experience dizziness or vertigo. However, with the addition of a new physiologic stressor, such as fever or hypoxia, they become acutely dizzy. Examples include patients with MS with fever from a urinary tract infection,[106] mild degenerative cerebellar ataxia with hypoxia from aspiration pneumonia, or remote posterior circulation stroke who have been started on a new sedative medication.[107]

Most neurologists are familiar with this phenomenon, sometimes referred to as unmasking prior symptoms or explained by the concept of the locus minoris resistentiae (point of least resistance). However, this phenomenon is poorly studied, and there is a dearth of medical literature on the subject. Two articles from the anesthesia literature describe patients with prior neurologic issues (stroke or tumor) who were carefully examined for neurologic deficits at baseline, then administered midazolam (with fentanyl in one of the studies), reexamined during the sedation, then examined a third time after the sedative effects had worn off.[108,109] The deficits included hemiparesis, aphasia, and hemineglect. Articles describing stroke mimics often ascribe cases ultimately diagnosed with systemic infection to this phenomenon; a prior history of stroke is a risk factor for this particular mimic.[107,110]

Recognizing this phenomenon is important for 2 reasons: (1) to understand that the primary issue is not an acute stroke and (2) to look for and treat the underlying physiologic stressor. This stressor may include fever, hypotension, hypoxia, medication effects, electrolyte or glucose abnormalities, and other toxic, metabolic, or infectious causes.

SUMMARY

For the emergency physician or specialist practicing in acute care settings, it is important to recognize that not all patients presenting with AVS have garden-variety vestibular neuritis or stroke. The differential diagnosis is broad, but most atypical cases have clear bedside clues that point to an uncommon, treatable cause (Table 1). Although most medical or other neurologic causes present no diagnostic confusion, frontline clinicians should have a high index of suspicion for certain rare disorders that require specific treatments and are easily missed, risking adverse consequences for patients.

Table 1
Special clues to suggest top 10 tricky causes of the acute vestibular syndrome requiring urgent, specific treatment (listed in order of descending urgency)

Condition	Clues	Initial Management
Wernicke syndrome	Malnutrition (especially bariatric surgery), combination of bilateral VOR deficits and gaze-evoked nystagmus	Intravenous thiamine Avoid glucose
Posterior fossa compartment syndrome	Headache, lethargy, hemiparesis; papilledema or sixth nerve palsies	Intubation/hyperventilation; ventriculostomy or posterior fossa surgical decompression Avoid lumbar puncture
Listeria rhombencephalitis	Recent febrile illness, abdominal pain, low-grade fever	Intravenous ampicillin Do not rely on cephalosporins
Carbon monoxide poisoning	Headache or confusion/lethargy; similarly affected individuals at home or work, including pets	Hyperbaric oxygen; secondary prevention of reexposure
Decompression sickness	History of diving or other decompressions	Hyperbaric oxygen; secondary prevention of reexposure
Ciguatera poisoning	Tropical travel, fish ingestion, circumoral paresthesia	Close observation of respiration, secondary prevention of reexposure
Miller Fisher syndrome	Ophthalmoplegia without obtundation, areflexia	Close observation of respiration, intravenous immunoglobulin
Bacterial labyrinthitis	History of surgical ear treatment, otalgia, or otorrhea; irritative nystagmus (toward the affected ear)	Intravenous antibiotics
Hypothyroidism/myxedema	Fatigue, weight gain, edema; hypothermia, bradycardia	Thyroid replacement
Paraneoplastic encephalitis	Severely affected patient with normal findings on MRI neuroimaging	Expedited workup for systemic malignancy; testicular cancer requires manual examination, ultrasonography Do not rely on PET-CT

Abbreviations: CT, computed tomography; VOR, vestibulo-ocular reflex.

ACKNOWLEDGMENTS

Dr. Newman-Toker's effort was supported, in part, by a grant from the National Institutes of Health, National Institute on Deafness and Other Communication Disorders (1U01DC013778-01A1).

REFERENCES

1. Newman-Toker DE, Hsieh YH, Camargo CA Jr, et al. Spectrum of dizziness visits to US emergency departments: cross-sectional analysis from a nationally representative sample. Mayo Clin Proc 2008;83:765–75.
2. Tarnutzer AA, Berkowitz AL, Robinson KA, et al. Does my dizzy patient have a stroke? A systematic review of bedside diagnosis in acute vestibular syndrome. CMAJ 2011;183:E571–92.

3. Maixner SM, Greden JF. Extended antidepressant maintenance and discontinuation syndromes. Depress Anxiety 1998;8(Suppl 1):43–53.

4. Maddox PT, Saunders J, Chandrasekhar SS. Sudden hearing loss from PDE-5 inhibitors: A possible cellular stress etiology. Laryngoscope 2009;119:1586–9.

5. Living without a balancing mechanism. N Engl J Med 1952;246:458–60.

6. Alekseeva N, McGee J, Kelley RE, et al. Toxic-metabolic, nutritional, and medicinal-induced disorders of cerebellum. Neurol Clin 2014;32:901–11.

7. Newman-Toker DE, Kattah JC, Alvernia JE, et al. Normal head impulse test differentiates acute cerebellar strokes from vestibular neuritis. Neurology 2008;70: 2378–85.

8. Seymour JF. Carbamazepine overdose. Features of 33 cases. Drug Saf 1993;8: 81–8.

9. Arbusow V, Strupp M, Brandt T. Amiodarone-induced severe prolonged head-positional vertigo and vomiting. Neurology 1998;51:917.

10. Fetter M, Haslwanter T, Bork M, et al. New insights into positional alcohol nystagmus using three-dimensional eye-movement analysis. Ann Neurol 1999; 45:216–23.

11. Ahmed RM, Hannigan IP, MacDougall HG, et al. Gentamicin ototoxicity: a 23-year selected case series of 103 patients. Med J Aust 2012;196:701–4.

12. Ariano RE, Zelenitsky SA, Kassum DA. Aminoglycoside-induced vestibular injury: maintaining a sense of balance. Ann Pharmacother 2008;42:1282–9.

13. Fava GA, Gatti A, Belaise C, et al. Withdrawal symptoms after selective serotonin reuptake inhibitor discontinuation: a systematic review. Psychother Psychosom 2015;84:72–81.

14. Blay SL. Nystagmus as a discontinuation symptom after antidepressant therapy: a case report. Prim Care Companion CNS Disord 2014;16 [pii: PCC.13l01615].

15. Smith PF, Darlington CL. A possible explanation for dizziness following SSRI discontinuation. Acta Otolaryngol 2010;130:981–3.

16. Meredith TJ, Ruprah M, Liddle A, et al. Diagnosis and treatment of acute poisoning with volatile substances. Hum Toxicol 1989;8:277–86.

17. He F, Wang S, Liu L, et al. Clinical manifestations and diagnosis of acute pyrethroid poisoning. Arch Toxicol 1989;63:54–8.

18. Bagnis R, Kuberski T, Laugier S. Clinical observations on 3,009 cases of ciguatera (fish poisoning) in the South Pacific. Am J Trop Med Hyg 1979;28:1067–73.

19. Heckerling PS, Leikin JB, Maturen A, et al. Predictors of occult carbon monoxide poisoning in patients with headache and dizziness. Ann Intern Med 1987;107: 174–6.

20. Daley WR, Smith A, Paz-Argandona E, et al. An outbreak of carbon monoxide poisoning after a major ice storm in Maine. J Emerg Med 2000;18:87–93.

21. Holt J, Weaver LK. Carbon monoxide poisoning mimicking arterial gas embolism in a commercial diver. Undersea Hyperb Med 2012;39:687–90.

22. Currier WD. Dizziness related to hypoglycemia: the role of adrenal steroids and nutrition. Laryngoscope 1971;81:18–35.

23. Weinger K, Jacobson AM, Draelos MT, et al. Blood glucose estimation and symptoms during hyperglycemia and hypoglycemia in patients with insulin-dependent diabetes mellitus. Am J Med 1995;98:22–31.

24. Jaap AJ, Jones GC, McCrimmon RJ, et al. Perceived symptoms of hypoglycaemia in elderly type 2 diabetic patients treated with insulin. Diabet Med 1998;15: 398–401.

25. Malouf R, Brust JC. Hypoglycemia: causes, neurological manifestations, and outcome. Ann Neurol 1985;17:421–30.

26. Warren RE, Deary IJ, Frier BM. The symptoms of hyperglycaemia in people with insulin-treated diabetes: classification using principal components analysis. Diabetes Metab Res Rev 2003;19:408–14.
27. Guisado R, Arieff AI. Neurologic manifestations of diabetic comas: correlation with biochemical alterations in the brain. Metabolism 1975;24:665–79.
28. Jahangiri A, Wagner J, Tran MT, et al. Factors predicting postoperative hyponatremia and efficacy of hyponatremia management strategies after more than 1000 pituitary operations. J Neurosurg 2013;119:1478–83.
29. Soupart A, Decaux G. Therapeutic recommendations for management of severe hyponatremia: current concepts on pathogenesis and prevention of neurologic complications. Clin Nephrol 1996;46:149–69.
30. Arieff AI, Guisado R. Effects on the central nervous system of hypernatremic and hyponatremic states. Kidney Int 1976;10:104–16.
31. Kumar S, Berl T. Sodium. Lancet 1998;352:220–8.
32. Bansal T, Abeygunasekara S, Ezzat V. An unusual presentation of primary renal hypokalemia-hypomagnesemia (Gitelman's syndrome). Ren Fail 2010;32:407–10.
33. Chon SB, Kwak YH, Hwang SS, et al. Severe hyperkalemia can be detected immediately by quantitative electrocardiography and clinical history in patients with symptomatic or extreme bradycardia: a retrospective cross-sectional study. J Crit Care 2013;28:1112.e7–13.
34. Grubina R, Klocke DL. 47-year-old woman with dizziness, weakness, and confusion. Mayo Clin Proc 2011;86:e1–4.
35. Ladenhauf HN, Stundner O, Spreitzhofer F, et al. Severe hyperphosphatemia after administration of sodium-phosphate containing laxatives in children: case series and systematic review of literature. Pediatr Surg Int 2012;28:805–14.
36. Lok U, Hatipoglu S, Gulacti U, et al. The role of thyroid and parathyroid metabolism disorders in the etiology of sudden onset dizziness. Med Sci Monit 2014;20:2689–94.
37. Lundberg E, Bergengren H, Lindqvist B. Mild phosphate diabetes in adults. Acta Med Scand 1978;204:93–6.
38. Satish R, Gokulnath G. Serum magnesium in recovering acute renal failure. Indian J Nephrol 2008;18:101–4.
39. Salomo LH, Laursen AH, Reiter N, et al. Myxoedema coma: an almost forgotten, yet still existing cause of multiorgan failure. BMJ Case Rep 2014;2014 [pii: bcr2013203223].
40. Stollberger C, Finsterer J, Brand E, et al. Dysarthria as the leading symptom of hypothyroidism. Am J Otolaryngol 2001;22:70–2.
41. Feit S, Feit H. Thyrotoxicosis factitia veterinarius. Ann Intern Med 1997;127:168.
42. Chen P, Chen HF, Tan SW, et al. Severely sustained vomiting as the main symptom in a man with thyrotoxicosis. J Chin Med Assoc 2003;66:311–4.
43. Bhatia PL, Gupta OP, Agrawal MK, et al. Audiological and vestibular function tests in hypothyroidism. Laryngoscope 1977;87:2082–9.
44. Crawford JR, Say D. Vitamin B12 deficiency presenting as acute ataxia. BMJ Case Rep 2013;2013 [pii: bcr2013008840].
45. Jayaram S, Soman A, Tarvade S, et al. Cerebellar ataxia due to isolated vitamin E deficiency. Indian J Med Sci 2005;59:20–3.
46. Galvin R, Brathen G, Ivashynka A, et al. EFNS guidelines for diagnosis, therapy and prevention of Wernicke encephalopathy. Eur J Neurol 2010;17:1408–18.
47. Kattah J, Dhanani S, Pula J. Vestibular signs of thiamine deficiency during the early phase of suspected Wernicke encephalopathy. Neurlogy Clinical Practice 2013;3:260–8.

48. Newman-Toker DE, Dy FJ, Stanton VA, et al. How often is dizziness from primary cardiovascular disease true vertigo? A systematic review. J Gen Intern Med 2008;23:2087–94.

49. Lasch KF, Evans CJ, Schatell D. A qualitative analysis of patient-reported symptoms of anemia. Nephrol Nurs J 2009;36:621–4, 631–2; [quiz: 33].

50. Abelsson J, Andreasson B, Samuelsson J, et al. Patients with polycythemia vera have worst impairment of quality of life among patients with newly diagnosed myeloproliferative neoplasms. Leuk Lymphoma 2013;54:2226–30.

51. Bodhit AN, Stead LG. Altered mental status and a not-so-benign rash. Case Rep Emerg Med 2011;2011:684572.

52. Kesler A, Ellis MH, Manor Y, et al. Neurological complications of essential thrombocytosis (ET). Acta Neurol Scand 2000;102:299–302.

53. Kwaan HC. Hyperviscosity in plasma cell dyscrasias. Clin Hemorheol Microcirc 2013;55:75–83.

54. Saito N, Watanabe M, Liao J, et al. Clinical and radiologic findings of inner ear involvement in sickle cell disease. AJNR Am J Neuroradiol 2011;32: 2160–4.

55. Sheth KJ, Swick HM, Haworth N. Neurological involvement in hemolytic-uremic syndrome. Ann Neurol 1986;19:90–3.

56. Hultcrantz E. Clinical treatment of vascular inner ear diseases. Am J Otolaryngol 1988;9:317–22.

57. Klingmann C. Inner ear decompression sickness in compressed-air diving. Undersea Hyperb Med 2012;39:589–94.

58. Swingler RJ, Compston DA. The morbidity of multiple sclerosis. Q J Med 1992; 83:325–37.

59. Pula JH, Newman-Toker DE, Kattah JC. Multiple sclerosis as a cause of the acute vestibular syndrome. J Neurol 2013;260:1649–54.

60. Sastre-Garriga J, Tintore M, Nos C, et al. Clinical features of CIS of the brainstem/cerebellum of the kind seen in MS. J Neurol 2010;257:742–6.

61. Zadro I, Barun B, Habek M, et al. Isolated cranial nerve palsies in multiple sclerosis. Clin Neurol Neurosurg 2008;110:886–8.

62. Frohman EM, Zhang H, Dewey RB, et al. Vertigo in MS: utility of positional and particle repositioning maneuvers. Neurology 2000;55:1566–9.

63. Gurol ME, St Louis EK. Treatment of cerebellar masses. Curr Treat Options Neurol 2008;10:138–50.

64. Javalkar V, Kelley RE, Gonzalez-Toledo E, et al. Acute ataxias: differential diagnosis and treatment approach. Neurol Clin 2014;32:881–91.

65. Park M, Kim K, Lee N, et al. The usefulness of MRI for acute isolated vertigo patients in the emergency department. Journal of International Advanced Otology 2014;10:162–6.

66. Pfiffner TJ, Jani R, Mechtler L. Neuro-oncological disorders of the cerebellum. Neurol Clin 2014;32:913–41.

67. Stark AM, Maslehaty H, Hugo HH, et al. Glioblastoma of the cerebellum and brainstem. J Clin Neurosci 2010;17:1248–51.

68. Behin A, Hoang-Xuan K, Carpentier AF, et al. Primary brain tumours in adults. Lancet 2003;361:323–31.

69. Omuro AM, Leite CC, Mokhtari K, et al. Pitfalls in the diagnosis of brain tumours. Lancet Neurol 2006;5:937–48.

70. Fadul C, Misulis KE, Wiley RG. Cerebellar metastases: diagnostic and management considerations. J Clin Oncol 1987;5:1107–15.

71. Zada G, Bond AE, Wang YP, et al. Incidence trends in the anatomic location of primary malignant brain tumors in the United States: 1992–2006. World Neurosurg 2012;77:518–24.
72. Brouwer MC, Coutinho JM, van de Beek D. Clinical characteristics and outcome of brain abscess: systematic review and meta-analysis. Neurology 2014;82: 806–13.
73. Yang SY. Brain abscess: a review of 400 cases. J Neurosurg 1981;55:794–9.
74. Brouwer MC, Tunkel AR, van de Beek D. Brain abscess. N Engl J Med 2014;371: 1758.
75. Honda H, Warren DK. Central nervous system infections: meningitis and brain abscess. Infect Dis Clin North Am 2009;23:609–23.
76. Singh TD, Fugate JE, Rabinstein AA. The spectrum of acute encephalitis: Causes, management, and predictors of outcome. Neurology 2015;84(4):359–66.
77. Moragas M, Martinez-Yelamos S, Majos C, et al. Rhombencephalitis: a series of 97 patients. Medicine 2011;90:256–61.
78. Jubelt B, Mihai C, Li TM, et al. Rhombencephalitis/brainstem encephalitis. Curr Neurol Neurosci Rep 2011;11:543–52.
79. Smiatacz T, Kowalik MM, Hlebowicz M. Prolonged dysphagia due to Listeria-rhombencephalitis with brainstem abscess and acute polyradiculoneuritis. J Infect 2006;52:e165–7.
80. Kaski D, Davies N, Seemungal BM. Varicella-zoster virus meningo-rhombencephalitis presenting as Ramsey Hunt. Neurology 2012;79:2291–2.
81. Philpot SJ, Archer JS. Herpes encephalitis preceded by ipsilateral vestibular neuronitis. J Clin Neurosci 2005;12:958–9.
82. Buki B, Tarnutzer A. Medical, non-vestibular causes of dizziness and vertigo. In: Vertigo and dizziness. Oxford (United Kingdom): Oxford University Press; 2014. p. 119–24.
83. Odaka M, Yuki N, Yamada M, et al. Bickerstaff's brainstem encephalitis: clinical features of 62 cases and a subgroup associated with Guillain-Barre syndrome. Brain 2003;126:2279–90.
84. Pruitt AA. Infections of the cerebellum. Neurol Clin 2014;32:1117–31.
85. Sawaishi Y, Takada G. Acute cerebellitis. Cerebellum 2002;1:223–8.
86. Cheung K, Fung H. An unusual case of dizziness presenting to emergency department: acute cerebellitis. Hong Kong J Emerg Med 2012;19:133–7.
87. Mantokoudis G, Saber Tehrani AS, Newman-Toker D. An unusual stroke-like clinical presentation of Creutzfeldt-Jacob disease: acute vestibular syndrome. Neurologist 2015;19(4):96–8.
88. Ko MW, Dalmau J, Galetta SL. Neuro-ophthalmologic manifestations of paraneoplastic syndromes. J Neuroophthalmol 2008;28:58–68.
89. Tafur AJ, Kreuziger LM, Quevedo F. 28-year-old man with severe vertigo. Mayo Clin Proc 2008;83:1070–3.
90. Kangsanarak J, Navacharoen N, Fooanant S, et al. Intracranial complications of suppurative otitis media: 13 years' experience. Am J Otol 1995;16:104–9.
91. Hyden D, Akerlind B, Peebo M. Inner ear and facial nerve complications of acute otitis media with focus on bacteriology and virology. Acta Otolaryngol 2006;126:460–6.
92. Ishizaki H, Pyykko I, Nozue M. Neuroborreliosis in the etiology of vestibular neuronitis. Acta Otolaryngol Suppl 1993;503:67–9.
93. Vercoe GS. The effect of early syphilis on the inner ear and auditory nerves. J Laryngol Otol 1976;90:853–61.

94. Jones JS, Nevai J, Freeman MP, et al. Emergency department presentation of idiopathic intracranial hypertension. Am J Emerg Med 1999;17:517–21.

95. Bruce BB, Lamirel C, Wright DW, et al. Nonmydriatic ocular fundus photography in the emergency department. N Engl J Med 2011;364:387–9.

96. Pons Y, Verillaud B, Ukkola-Pons E, et al. Pulsatile tinnitus and venous cerebral thrombosis: report of a case and literature review. Rev Laryngol Otol Rhinol (Bord) 2012;133:163–4.

97. Gameiro J, Ferro JM, Canhao P, et al. Prognosis of cerebral vein thrombosis presenting as isolated headache: early vs. late diagnosis. Cephalalgia 2012;32:407–12.

98. Mehrenberger M, Kamar N, Borde JS, et al. Vertigo after renal transplantation: a sign of paucisymptomatic cryptococcal meningitis. Exp Clin Transplant 2006;4:525–7.

99. Lamy C, Oppenheim C, Mas JL. Posterior reversible encephalopathy syndrome. Handb Clin Neurol 2014;121:1687–701.

100. Schwartz RB. Hyperperfusion encephalopathies: hypertensive encephalopathy and related conditions. Neurologist 2002;8:22–34.

101. Maggiorini M, Buhler B, Walter M, et al. Prevalence of acute mountain sickness in the Swiss Alps. BMJ 1990;301:853–5.

102. Shintani S, Hino T, Ishihara S, et al. Reversible brainstem hypertensive encephalopathy (RBHE): Clinicoradiologic dissociation. Clin Neurol Neurosurg 2008;110:1047–53.

103. Salkic S, Batic-Mujanovic O, Ljuca F, et al. Clinical presentation of hypertensive crises in emergency medical services. Mater Sociomed 2014;26:12–6.

104. Yang WC, Wu HP. Clinical analysis of hypertension in children admitted to the emergency department. Pediatr Neonatol 2010;51:44–51.

105. Isildak H, Albayram S, Isildak H. Spontaneous intracranial hypotension syndrome accompanied by bilateral hearing loss and venous engorgement in the internal acoustic canal and positional change of audiography. J Craniofac Surg 2010;21:165–7.

106. Mahadeva A, Tanasescu R, Gran B. Urinary tract infections in multiple sclerosis: under-diagnosed and under-treated? A clinical audit at a large university hospital. Am J Clin Exp Immunol 2014;3:57–67.

107. Tobin WO, Hentz JG, Bobrow BJ, et al. Identification of stroke mimics in the emergency department setting. J Brain Dis 2009;1:19–22.

108. Lazar RM, Fitzsimmons BF, Marshall RS, et al. Reemergence of stroke deficits with midazolam challenge. Stroke 2002;33:283–5.

109. Thal GD, Szabo MD, Lopez-Bresnahan M, et al. Exacerbation or unmasking of focal neurologic deficits by sedatives. Anesthesiology 1996;85:21–5 [discussion: 29A–30A].

110. Libman RB, Wirkowski E, Alvir J, et al. Conditions that mimic stroke in the emergency department. Implications for acute stroke trials. Arch Neurol 1995;52:1119–22.

111. Ullman E, Edlow JA. Complete heart block complicating the head impulse test. Arch Neurol 2010;67:1272–4.

112. Newman-Toker DE, Kerber KA, Hsieh YH, et al. HINTS outperforms ABCD2 to screen for stroke in acute continuous vertigo and dizziness. Acad Emerg Med 2013;20:986–96.

Index

Note: Page numbers of article titles are in **boldface** type.

Neurol Clin 33 (2015) 717–725
http://dx.doi.org/10.1016/S0733-8619(15)00054-7
0733-8619/15/$ – see front matter © 2015 Elsevier Inc. All rights reserved.

neurologic.theclinics.com

Printed and bound by CPI Group (UK) Ltd, Croydon, CR0 4YY

18/10/2024

01775941-0003